Managing
the Injured
Athlete

Commissioning Editor: Rita Demetriou-Swanwick
Development Editor: Veronika Watkins
Project Manager: Gopika Sasidharan/Divya Krish
Designer: Charles Gray
Illustration Manager: Gillian Richards

Managing the Injured Athlete

Assessment, Rehabilitation and Return to Play

Written by

Zoë Hudson PhD, MCSP

Honorary Senior Clinical Lecturer, Centre for Sports and Exercise Medicine, Barts and the London School of Medicine and Dentistry, Queen Mary University of London
Editor, Physical Therapy in Sport

Claire Small MPhty St., MMACP

Clinical Director, Pure Sports Medicine, London
Honorary Clinical Lecturer, Center for Sports and Exercise Medicine, Barts and the London School of Medicine and Dentistry, Queen Mary University of London

Edinburgh   London   New York   Oxford   Philadelphia   St Louis   Sydney   Toronto   2011

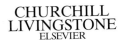

CHURCHILL
LIVINGSTONE
ELSEVIER

© 2011 Elsevier Ltd. All rights reserved.

ISBN 978-0-7020-3004-8

British Library Cataloguing in Publication Data
A catalogue record for this book is available from the British Library

Library of Congress Cataloging in Publication Data
A catalog record for this book is available from the Library of Congress

Notices
Knowledge and best practice in this field are constantly changing. As new research and experience broaden our understanding, changes in research methods, professional practices, or medical treatment may become necessary.

Practitioners and researchers must always rely on their own experience and knowledge in evaluating and using any information, methods, compounds, or experiments described herein. In using such information or methods they should be mindful of their own safety and the safety of others, including parties for whom they have a professional responsibility.

With respect to any drug or pharmaceutical products identified, readers are advised to check the most current information provided (i) on procedures featured or (ii) by the manufacturer of each product to be administered, to verify the recommended dose or formula, the method and duration of administration, and contraindications. It is the responsibility of practitioners, relying on their own experience and knowledge of their patients, to make diagnoses, to determine dosages and the best treatment for each individual patient, and to take all appropriate safety precautions.

To the fullest extent of the law, neither the Publisher nor the authors, contributors, or editors, assume any liability for any injury and/or damage to persons or property as a matter of products liability, negligence or otherwise, or from any use or operation of any methods, products, instructions, or ideas contained in the material herein.

ELSEVIER your source for books,
journals and multimedia
in the health sciences

www.elsevierhealth.com

Working together to grow
libraries in developing countries

www.elsevier.com | www.bookaid.org | www.sabre.org

ELSEVIER   BOOK AID
International   Sabre Foundation

The
Publisher's
policy is to use
**paper manufactured
from sustainable forests**

Printed in China

CONTENTS

Foreword

In my experience the most difficult question you are faced with when working in competitive sport is whether an individual can race or return to the field of play during training or major competition after the onset of an injury. This can be a real challenge, and sometimes is career changing for the athlete in question. There is no definitive answer and often you have no one with whom you can discuss your reasoning. You are considered the expert and you will have to live with the consequences of the judgement you make. You will on occasions watch anxiously the player you have sent back out into the field of play wondering if you took the right judgement, you will lose sleep, and you will share in the jubilation when your decision brings the sought reward. With time your own experience will allow you to develop your clinical reasoning for situations that arise commonly within the sport that you are associated with, however there will always be presentations that do not quite make sense. A pocket book of this nature will help you to unravel these clinical conundrums.

This book is a welcome and long overdue addition to the increasing resources available in the still evolving field of Sports Medicine. It is a very practical pocket book that provides a framework from which anyone working in sport could determine the most likely diagnosis for a clinical presentation and the most appropriate treatment/activity protocol. A prerequisite for every sports team medical bag.

Dr Ann Redgrave BSc, MBBS, DO, MSc SEM.
Chief Medical Officer GB Rowing Team

Acknowledgements

As clinicians, educators and researchers, in this book we have drawn on information gathered from several sources and owe many thanks to them all for this. Our patients, whose clinical experiences have informed us about different presentations of pathology and different responses to treatment, have taught us to be innovative and reflective in our assessment and management. Our students have challenged our teaching and communication processes, helping us develop different ways of imparting knowledge and facilitating skills in evaluative thinking, patient handling and treatment. And our clinical colleagues from whom we have "stolen" clever manual techniques and rehabilitation exercises, discussed countless "problem" patients, watched managing new or unfamiliar conditions, seen operate, inject and image and heard present on specialist topics. Our thanks to all these people whose experiences and expertise have helped shape this book.

Thanks also to the team at Elsevier, Rita Demetriou-Swanwick and Veronika Watkins, who nudged us along throughout the project, encouraging us to focus and complete this book on top of our existing workloads.

To Mark Slocombe from Creation Video and our models Alex and Michael for their work on the photographs. Working with two physios with perfectionist tendencies often meant taking the same image several times to get the right shot. However, we think the results were worth the effort.

And finally to our family and friends, our thanks for their enthusiastic support and their encouragement to see this text completed.

Acknowledgements

The following pictures in this book have been taken from: McDonald: Pocketbook of Taping Techniques, reproduced with permission of Elsevier: 1.1a, 1.1b, 1.1c, 1.2a, 1.2b, 1.3a, 1.3b, 1.4a, 1.4b, 1.5a, 1.5b, 1.5c, 1.6a, 1.6b, 1.6c, 1.6d, 3.3a, 3.3b, 3.3c, 3.3d.

The following pictures have been taken from Hewetson: An Illustrated Guide to Taping Techniques: 3.2a, 3.2b – and 2.29, 2.37 and 2.46 from Pope: Imaging of the Musculoskeletal System, Vol 1, reproduced with permission of Elsevier.

Introduction

This pocketbook is aimed at all those clinicians who are working, or are aiming to work, with teams or individual athletes and is relevant to clinicians working in the field of musculoskeletal medicine. It is a pocketbook and not a textbook, and as such, it is small enough to be thrown into your medical bag for quick reference out in the field if needed.

In addition to the usual sections (assessment, treatment and rehabilitation) that you would expect to see in this book, there are sections dealing with your role working within a team, athlete confidentiality, travelling with athletes, drugs and doping issues, working in different climates and return-to-play considerations. These are important issues and your success will be determined not just by your clinical skills, but also by how you deal with your working environment and all the other issues within this.

We have been teaching at undergraduate and postgraduate level for many years and we share a similar philosophy. You can teach anyone manual techniques or exercise prescription, and whilst excellent hands-on skills and innovative exercise prescription are essential, the real skill is knowing when to deploy these techniques. Developing good clinical reasoning skills is critical in becoming a good clinician. Identifying patterns of clinical presentation is the key to problem solving and formulating a "diagnosis". In the field of clinical reasoning this has been recognised as the process most commonly employed by expert clinicians. Sometimes these clinical patterns can be fairly predictable, as in the case of a simple ankle sprain; however, in the case of something such as groin pain, these patterns can be very inconsistent and less easily distinguished. Equally, some less common pathologies can have clinical findings that are very similar to more commonly seen conditions. Clinicians who have less clinical mileage can find it difficult to identify these more unusual conditions, as they are not pathologies or presentations that they have encountered. In these "cases of the unknown", it is not unusual for any clinician to make incorrect diagnoses. It would be like hearing hoof beats and assuming it is a horse, when actually the same sounds may be coming from a zebra – similar in many ways, but an entirely different creature!

Ensuring you have not missed a less common condition is extremely important, as some pathologies have only a limited "window of opportunity" to be managed appropriately. This is especially relevant if you are working single-handed in a club where a second opinion may not be readily available.

We have written Section 2 on Assessment with this in mind. As well as providing guidelines for assessment of the spine and periphery, we have detailed the subjective and physical examination findings for numerous clinical conditions. Unfortunately, research information regarding clinical presentations is extremely limited, so we have also drawn on our years of clinical practice to describe these conditions. To assist diagnostic decision making, we have developed a key to indicate how frequently clinicians can expect to come across certain subjective and objective markers for a given condition. We have used the format below and hope this assists in the clinical reasoning process.

Patterns of positive findings:

✓✓✓	Nearly always
✓✓	Often
✓	Sometimes

In Section 3, we present the underlying principles of injury rehabilitation with a series of case studies to demonstrate how these can be put into practice. These case studies are not to be used as "recipe-style" rehabilitation programmes, but rather to illustrate the goal-driven principles that we advocate and help the clinician translate their patient-specific goals into a suitable rehabilitation programme. Every individual athlete will present and respond to treatment slightly differently and any rehabilitation programme needs to be adjusted accordingly.

We have also introduced several other features in an attempt to make this book as clinically useful as possible:

 Clinical tips: The light bulb indicates any top clinical tips that we think would be helpful or that are important to consider in management.

 Evidence: We live in a world of evidence-based medicine and we have used the tick symbol to indicate where there is good evidence available in the literature to support the intervention described. It is important for clinicians to recognize where good evidence does exist for our management strategies. But it is equally important to remember that little or no evidence to support an intervention does not mean that we should not use the treatment. It may simply mean that the research required is currently too complex or too invasive to undertake. Utilizing good validated outcome measures with our patients and noting the effects of our interventions on these measures is an effective way of performing clinical research every day.

 Further reading: There are no lists of references at the end of each section as this book is focused primarily on clinical practice and the reader can refer to other "textbooks" for more detailed information and references on a topic. However, we have highlighted some specific research papers that readers can refer to for more information.

We have worked in the fields of sports and musculoskeletal medicine for long enough to recognize that clinicians of all levels of experience are often working as sole practitioners. This can be in very isolated club or competition environments with limited support or opportunity to discuss clinical problems. Our aim with this pocketbook is to provide support, to help answer clinical queries and solve clinical problems when there may be no-one else to refer to.

Working in sport often throws up situations that weren't covered in university or college lectures or in the in-service training at the hospital. We have therefore tried to put down on paper information that, over time, we have found valuable. Some of this has been learnt first hand, some has come as advice from athletes, coaches and managers, and much of it has been passed on by other, more experienced, clinicians with whom we have worked. We hope you find it valuable, whether as new information to a new practitioner or as an aide memoire to those of you who have been practising for several years.

Zoe Hudson & Claire Small
London, April 2011

Working in sport

Introduction

Working with a team or individual athletes can be one of the most rewarding aspects of a clinician's career, but also one of the most demanding. Competition environments are often extremely stressful and it is not unusual for the pitchside clinician to find themselves in unfamiliar territory dealing with an unaccustomed injury or situation. This section is designed to familiarize the clinician with fundamental elements and skills associated with working in a sporting environment, and to highlight key areas for development.

Know your role

It is essential that all pitchside clinicians safeguard themselves by working only within the scope of practice in which they feel competent. In the world of modern medicine, scope of practice is rarely rigidly defined for any profession, be they a doctor, physiotherapist, sports therapist or osteopath. Professional bodies and the legal system have recognized the importance of avoiding restrictive boundaries for practice, as to do so may limit the professional development of the individual.

While this is advantageous in many team scenarios where one clinician is often expected to wear the hats of many professions, it also places the onus for clinical decision-making and action squarely on the clinician's shoulders. Before undertaking any clinical decision or activity, the clinician must always ask themselves, "Do I feel competent to do this?".

The question of competency is more than simply, "Have I done a course or workshop which qualifies me to do this?". It is also about undertaking these practices on a regular basis and under similar circumstances, and reflecting on and reviewing your clinical practice with peers and as an individual. Clinicians should refer to their professional bodies (www.csp.org.uk, www.osteopathy.org.uk, www.basrat.org, www.bma.org.uk) for information and guidance on scope of practice specific to their profession.

It is important to recognize that you are responsible for the team you are working with. In the event of an injury, it is your decisions which are important. Do not let yourself be influenced by the comments or opinions of spectators or players, no matter what their qualifications are.

Sometimes, student physiotherapists are approached to act as team physiotherapists for amateur clubs and organizations that struggle to find or fund a qualified physiotherapist. It is essential for student physiotherapists to be aware that under the terms of the Chartered Society of Physiotherapy (CSP)'s Professional Liability Insurance (PLI) they are only insured to practise both within their own level of competence and **under the supervision of a qualified physiotherapist.**

Likewise, qualified physiotherapists sometimes find themselves working alongside students to cover events and tournaments. If they are not happy to take on the responsibility of supervising students in this situation, this needs to be made clear to the organizers and alternative arrangements should be discussed. Having responsibility for students does not mean taking responsibility for any mistakes, but it does mean understanding the students' level of competency and ensuring they are expected to practise only within these limits, as would be the case in a clinical setting.

In addition, the opposition team should never be relied on to provide medical support, as the level of cover may very well be insufficient or inadequate.

In recent years, sport has become an increasingly litigious arena. Clinicians need to be mindful that actions which contravene the rules and codes of the sport they are covering may actually also have legal ramifications and/or place their professional registration in jeopardy.

Know your sport

Confidence in dealing with any situation improves with familiarity. If you are unfamiliar with a sport you are covering it is worth reading up on or discussing with a knowledgeable individual the nature and nuances of the game, the various positions played and the specific demands of these. It is also worthwhile discussing the physical demands and likely injuries with a colleague who has worked in the sport.

If you are working with a sport that is conducted in unusual settings, such as ice skating, skiing, swimming or sailing, special consideration for dealing with injuries, retrievals and evacuations is necessary to ensure you are prepared for these possibilities.

For physiotherapists serious about developing a role within professional sport some national bodies have a structured accreditation process. For example, in the UK the Association of Chartered Physiotherapists in Sports Medicine (ACPSM; www.acpsm.org) has a process in place that incorporates mentorship. Elements of the continuing professional development process include shadowing and observation.

It is not always necessary for your mentor to be involved in the same sport that you are working in; however, as some scenarios and the rules governing them are very sport specific it is worthwhile spending some time with more experienced people working in the same sport.

Scenarios and rules that are specific to certain sports include:

- Dealing with a blood injury – does the player need to leave the field? Can they return to the field of play?
- Treating an injury on/off field – can a player leave the field/court for treatment and return?
- Are substitutions permitted for injuries?
- Is the trainer permitted into the field of play to assess an injury and for how long? For example, in tennis, the trainer must be escorted onto the court by an official. They are permitted as long as necessary for assessment of the injured player but only 3 minutes for treatment once a diagnosis has been made.
- Similarly, Judo has several rules governing medical disqualifications and the presence of medical staff on the mat.

- Many organizations also have specific rules governing a player's return to competition following a head injury/concussion.

As well as discussing these rules with fellow clinicians and coaching staff, the governing bodies of each sport should be able to provide you with detailed information.

Working alone with a team can be difficult as you have no-one to discuss clinical scenarios with. Finding a mentor that you can speak and meet with regularly is an excellent method of improving your clinical skills. Utilizing web-based resources such as the British Association of Sport and Exercise Medicine (BASEM) forum (www.basem.co.uk) interactive CSP for physiotherapists (www.interactivecsp.org.uk), BASRaT (www.basrat.org), the British Osteopathic Association (www.osteopathy.org) and the Neuro Orthopaedic Institute (NOI; www.noigroup.com) provides even the most isolated clinician with access to other professionals working in the field of sports and musculoskeletal medicine.

Know your team

When starting work with a team, it is invaluable to spend time taking a detailed medical and sporting profile from all athletes. This allows you to determine the need for any preventative management and treatment, and to identify any athlete with special requirements or those who may be more vulnerable to illness or injury while competing. The information may also be invaluable in the event of an emergency when an athlete requires urgent medical care or transfer to hospital.

Form 1.1 provides a list of recommended information clinicians should obtain from all their players. This information should be documented as a confidential record, available at all training sessions and events. Access to the information should be limited to the medical team and head coaching staff. It must be signed by the player as an accurate record of their health status. In the event that they are under the age of 18, a parent or legal guardian is required to sign the form.

Form 1.1 Medical screening information

Confidential medical information

Name: . . . .

DOB: . . . .

Sex: . . . .

Height: . . . .   Weight: . . . .

Blood type: (Amenable to transfusions? Y/N) . . . .

Address and contact details: . . . .
. . . .
. . . .

Occupation: . . . .

Emergency contact details (including relationship to athlete): . . . .
. . . .
. . . .

GP's contact details: . . . .
. . . .
. . . .

Dentist's contact details: . . . .
. . . .
. . . .

Physiotherapist's contact details: . . . .
. . . .
. . . .

Private insurance details (if any): . . . .
. . . .
. . . .

Pre-existing medical conditions (including allergies): . . . .
. . . .
. . . .

Medication (including supplements): . . . .
. . . .
. . . .

Past history – musculoskeletal conditions (plus any residual problems): .
. . . .
. . . .

Any history of:
- ❏ Heart disease/condition
- ❏ Epilepsy
- ❏ Diabetes
- ❏ Asthma
- ❏ Dizziness
- ❏ Loss of consciousness
- ❏ Head injury/concussion
- ❏ Chest pain
- ❏ Fractures
- ❏ Dislocations

Existing injuries (current management):
. . . .
. . . .
. . . .

Family history (diabetes/heart disease/arthritic conditions):
. . . .
. . . .
. . . .

Personal habits:
- ❏ Smoking
- ❏ Alcohol
- ❏ Recreational drugs
- ❏ Diet and nutrition
- ❏ Hydration

Hep B status:
. . . .
. . . .

Tetanus status:

. . . .
. . . .

HIV status:

. . . .
. . . .

Female athlete-specific questions:

❏ Age at which menstruation started
❏ Regularity of menstrual cycles
❏ Use of oral contraceptive pills

Sporting history

Level of competition played:

. . . .
. . . .

Number of years at this level:

. . . .
. . . .

Position played:

. . . .
. . . .

Training hours per week: – This season
                           – Last season
Playing hours per week: – This season
                           – Last season

Do you wear glasses or contact lenses (specify)?:

Protective equipment:

❏ Brace
❏ Tape
❏ Mouthguard
❏ Helmet

Player signature: **Date:**

All professional organizations and high-level athletes together with many serious amateur teams and individuals will undergo some sort of musculoskeletal screening in pre-season, with the aim of implementing "pre-hab" programmes to prevent injury and enhance performance. The make-up and extent of these screenings is specific to the individual sports and is based on the sporting requirements and competition level.

At present, there is little supporting evidence that current musculoskeletal screening programmes predict or prevent re-injury in sport. Many organizations are therefore moving away from static and non-functional assessments of joint range and muscle strength towards functionally-based programmes that assess a player's ability to perform a variety of tasks that demand differing joint ranges and elements of muscle strength and control during multi-joint movements. Examples of the types of movement screened in this way include squats and lunges with rotation. It is hoped that future research will show the benefit of these more functional screenings in predicting and preventing injury.

Know your location

Whether you are working with athletes competing at home or abroad, preparatory research into the location of the competition will ensure you are able to deal with any injury or illness in the most efficient and effective way.

Prior to arriving at the venue, you should establish the location and facilities available at the nearest hospital, including the presence of an A&E department. You should also find out the likely transit time to and from the hospital, so that, in the event of an injury, you know how long you may have to manage the situation without ambulance support. In more isolated areas or less developed countries, there may be some time between calling for an ambulance and its arrival.

It is also worthwhile knowing the number for the hospital switchboard to inform them of any serious injuries.

You no doubt know the number for the emergency services in your own country, but it is possible that it is not the same number if you are abroad. Establish what the emergency number is in the country you are visiting.

In the event that an ambulance is required, you should be able to provide the emergency operator with information about accessing the sporting field or arena. Many sporting competitions are large events with several locations. Specific details regarding your location within the event, as well as the closest access points, will be helpful in an emergency situation. In the case of large events, the organizers will usually have provided the local hospital and ambulance service with details of the competition and will have established procedures for dealing with injuries. It is important to have knowledge of these procedures and the organizer's contact details to inform them if a serious injury occurs.

When you arrive at a venue, you, or someone designated by you, should check the arena/pitch or court for any potential hazards. These can include broken glass and other rubbish, dog dirt or excess water. Clearing the pitch or court of all hazards is not always possible, and if this is the case, the safety of the venue should be discussed.

You should also locate any medical facilities and the equipment stored within (Box 1.1). In many amateur events, the medical facilities are usually far from ideal. You should never expect to have access to any facilities or equipment that you do not carry yourself.

At many sporting events, no medical room will be available. In these instances, injuries need to be addressed on the side of the field. Make sure you move any injured player a sufficient distance from the field of play to protect them from the risk of further injury and allow adequate room for treatment and ambulance access if required.

Know your kit bag

The most important thing about your kit bag is that you know exactly what it contains and what each item is used for. The exact content of your kit bag will depend on your

Box 1.1   Provisions for a first aid room

- KEY – gaining access
- Telephone
- List of emergency contact numbers and procedures posted next to the telephone
- First aid kit
- Sink with hot and cold water available
- Disposable hand towels and liquid soap
- Towels
- Antiseptic gel
- Examination couch with pillows and blankets
- Chairs
- Lockable cupboard for records and drugs
- Separate containers for sharps/contaminated waste and general rubbish
- Access to electrical power supply
- Access to refrigeration for ice/cold packs/medical supplies
- Clock with a second hand
- Resuscitation equipment – pocket mask ± Ambu bag (bag valve mask, BVM)
- Defibrillator – requires qualified personnel

level of competency and training. You should not carry any item you are not trained or do not feel competent to use.

Do not let other people tamper with your bag. Items should be stored in and returned to the same place each time, so that an item is readily to hand when you need it urgently.

Your kit bag should be:

- Lightweight
- Portable
- Waterproof
- Durable
- Compartmentalized

Within your kit bag, clear plastic containers or plastic zip-lock bags are a useful way of keeping things well separated and easily identifiable. Bags and containers also protect items should you have an unexpected spill or leak. Zip-lock plastic bags also make useful ice packs.

Working in sport

Recommendations for a kit bag are listed in Table 1.1. To make up a kit bag for the sport or activity you are covering, select those items that are necessary to manage the types of injury that occur most commonly. It is always worthwhile discussing this with a colleague who works with the same sport to ensure you have not overlooked anything.

Table 1.1 Recommendations for a basic kit bag

Taping/strapping and management of soft tissue injuries	Use
Tape scissors	Cutting tape/removal of tape or clothing
Safety scissors	For cutting foam/adhesive
Zinc oxide tape in 2 sizes – 25 and 38 mm	Taping knees/shoulders / wrists and ankles
Elasticized crepe bandages	Apply compression to joints and limit oedema
Elastic cohesive bandages – various sizes	Apply support to joints
Elastic adhesive bandages (EAB) – 5 and 7.5 cm	
Ice/ice packs	Prevention of bleeding/swelling
Underwrap	For sensitive skin
Adhesive foam or felt	To assist compression or provide protection for bony areas
Tape adhesive spray/gel	To assist tape adherence and protect skin

Management of wounds	Use
Disposable nitrile gloves	Maintaining universal precautions
Gauze swabs	Swabbing wounds and applying creams and lotions
Adhesive dressings	Wound dressing
Sterile/non-adhesive dressings (various sizes)	Covering and protecting wounds of various sizes
Band-Aids – waterproof/non-allergenic	Covering small/minor wounds
Betadine	Cleaning antiseptic
Steri-Strips	Bring edges of wounds together

(Continued)

12

Table 1.1 Recommendations for a basic kit bag—cont'd

Management of wounds	Use
Tweezers (disposable or sterilized after use)	Removal of wound debris
Sterile needles/blood lancets	Wound management/removal of foreign bodies/blisters
Syringes	Wound irrigation
Sterile solution	Wound irrigation
Gauze bandages	Securing wound dressings in place
Micropore tape	Securing bandages and dressings
Alcohol swabs	Cleaning equipment/prior to needle use on unpunctured skin

Splints and braces	
Triangular bandages	Arm slings/splints/broad bandages

Other items	
Injury record forms	Recording injuries in a consistent manner
Pen and paper	
Resuscitation mask	Maintaining universal precautions
Defibrillator	Restoring normal circulation (must be certified in using this equipment)
Rigid cervical collar (several sizes required)	Management of spinal injury – used in conjunction with a spinal board
Oropharyngeal airway	Airway maintenance
Nasopharyngeal airway	Airway maintenance

Sports/player-specific items	
Shorts	Any item prescribed specifically for a player must be obtained by them from their doctor or pharmacist. However, if you are the only medical staff present, it falls to you to be responsible for carrying the medication during the event. You should discuss administration with the player prior to the event
Spare studs and screwdriver	
Spare shoelaces	
Mirror	
Contact lenses	
Prescribed medication	
– Inhalers	
– EpiPen®	
Glucose tablets	Hypoglycaemia

From Sports Medicine Australia.

It is common for some drugs and equipment to remain unused in a kit bag for some time. You should check all items for expiry dates on a regular basis and replace if necessary.

Know your Strapping

The extent to which strapping is utilized in any given sport depends on both the nature of the sport and the nature of the participants. As previously discussed, it is essential that you know your sport to ensure that any strapping you apply to a player does not contravene the rules of the sport and thus make the player ineligible to play. If you are considering strapping a player on the field, you need to ensure there is adequate time for this. A good example is an injury break in a tennis match where the trainer/clinician has only 3 minutes to complete the necessary treatment. In these instances, having the tape pre-torn speeds up the process and ensures the taping achieves its objectives.

Some guidelines for the application of tape:

- Encourage the player to shave the area to be taped
- Ask the player if they are aware of any allergies to tape or adhesives
- Apply adhesive spray to ensure better tape adhesion and protect the skin
- Consider whether felt or foam padding is required to protect exposed or bony regions

- Never tape a player for competition if the strapping technique has not been trialled in training and found to be effective

Underwrap – yes or no?

Underwrap is used in some cases to protect sensitive skin. Whether it is used depends upon the preferences of both the clinician and the player. Many clinicians find it makes effective support and stability of the joint difficult to achieve initially, and that during play it loosens easily and quickly becomes ineffective. However, the research evidence does not support this notion and it may well be that therapists feel more confident and are more technically proficient in the strapping techniques they are used to, whether this is with or without underwrap. Some players prefer the use of underwrap, as it is more comfortable and results in minimal skin irritation.

Similarly little evidence exists to support the use of preventative or prophylactic strapping in many sporting activities. One exception is the use of an external support (bracing or strapping) following ligamentous injury of the ankle reduces the risk of re-injury.

When discussing strapping with players, you should raise the prospect that a strapped joint or region may be considered "target practice" by the opposition as an indication of a potential weakness. Some players elect to strap the regions bilaterally in an attempt to confuse their opponent.

The following section covers some of the more commonly used strapping techniques in sports medicine.

Thumb spica

Aim: to provide support for the 1st metacarpophalangeal (MCP) joint.

Tape: 2.5 cm adhesive zinc oxide tape.

Application:
- Apply an anchor strap around the wrist
- Starting on the ulnar side of the wrist, take the 1st piece of tape over the dorsum of the hand and across the lateral joint line (Fig 1.1a). Continue around the thumb over the medial joint line, down across the palmar aspect of the hand to the starting point (Fig 1.1b)
- Repeat with further strips, covering the previous layer by 50% until adequate stability is achieved
- Apply an anchor strip over the wrist to hold the strapping in place (Fig 1.1c)

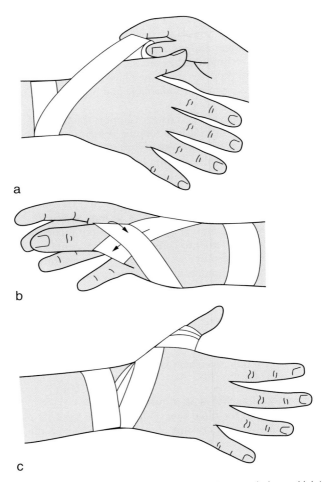

a

b

c

Fig 1.1 Thumb spica to support the 1st metacarpophalangeal joint showing (a) lateral joint support, (b) medial joint support and (c) completed taping.

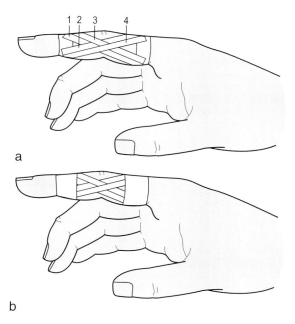

Fig 1.2 Finger tape to support the collateral ligaments (medial and lateral) showing (a) support for the lateral collateral and (b) completed taping.

Finger splinting

Fingers can be taped together in a buddy system by taping over the phalanges (not the joints) using 2.5 cm tape. Place a strip of foam between the fingers to support the injured finger.

Aim: To support the collateral ligaments of a single finger.

Tape: 2.5 cm adhesive zinc oxide tape torn in half to create 1.25 cm strips.

Application:
• Apply an anchor tape around both the middle and proximal phalanges

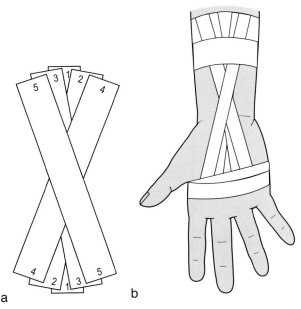

Fig 1.3 Strapping to support a wrist sprain and limit motion showing (a) fan of tape applied to either the dorsal surface of the forearm to control flexion or the palmar surface to control extension and (b) completed taping.

- Apply a strip of tape from the dorsal/medial aspect of the middle phalanx to the palmar/lateral aspect of the proximal phalanx
- Cover this with a strip running from the palmar/lateral aspect of the middle phalanx to the dorsal/medial aspect of the proximal phalanx, crossing the first tape at the level of the lateral joint line. Repeat with 2 further strips of tape (Fig 1.2a)
- Repeat on the medial side of the joint and then apply anchor straps to the middle and proximal phalanges (Fig 1.2b)

Wrist strapping

Aim: To support a sprained wrist and limit movement.

Tape: 2.5 cm adhesive zinc oxide tape.

Application:

- Apply 2 anchor tapes – one across the middle of the hand and the other in the mid forearm region
- Apply a fan of tape to either the dorsal or palmar aspect of the wrist depending on whether you are trying to control flexion or extension (Fig 1.3a)
- Lock the fan of tape in place by repeating the anchor strips (Fig 1.3b)
- TIP: Place the wrist in a slightly flexed position when taping to control extension, and vice versa

A similar taping technique can also be used at the elbow to control or limit extension.

Shoulder

Aim: This technique may elevate the shoulder and support the AC joint. Many players of contact sports like to have their shoulders taped prophylactically, thinking that this will help avoid dislocation. The clinician will recognize that this taping technique will not mechanically prevent this, but may influence proprioception.

Tape: 3.8 cm adhesive zinc oxide tape.

Application:

- The player sits with the elbow supported to maintain the shoulder in an elevated position
- Apply 2 anchor strips to the arm just below the deltoid tuberosity
- Apply a strip of tape from the anterior arm, up over the AC joint and posteriorly to finish at the level of the scapular spine
- Apply a 2nd strip from the posterior arm, up over the posterior acromion to finish over the AC joint (Fig 1.4a)

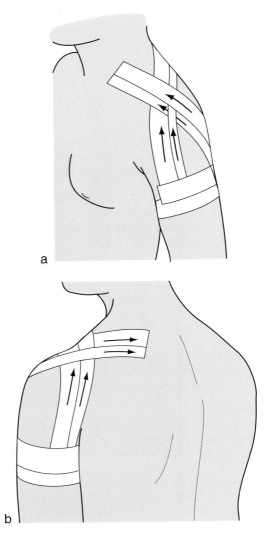

a

b

Fig 1.4 Shoulder taping to support the AC joint: (a) anterior view and (b) posterior view of overlapping strips.

- Repeat these 2 steps in an overlapping fashion until the player and clinician are satisfied that support is adequate (Fig 1.4b)
- Finish with an anchor strip around the arm to lock the tape in place

Ankle

Aim: to support the ankle following an inversion sprain.

Tape: 3.8 cm adhesive zinc oxide tape.

Application:
- Applied with the foot dorsiflexed and everted
- Apply an anchor at the level of the midfoot
- Apply a 2nd anchor to the shin about 10 cm above the malleoli (Fig 1.5a)
- Apply the vertical stirrup starting at the medial aspect of the shin anchor. Take the tape inferiorly over the medial malleolus, under the heel and pull firmly up on the

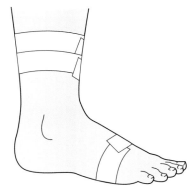

a

Fig 1.5 Tape for an inversion sprain of the ankle showing (a) anchor strips,

(Continued)

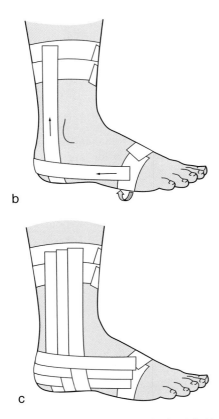

b

c

Fig 1.5—cont'd (b) vertical stirrups and horizontal strips, and (c) over lapping vertical stirrups and horizontal strips to produce a basketweave effect.

lateral aspect, over the lateral malleolus, to attach to the lateral shin anchor
- **Do not conform the tape to the leg**
- Apply the horizontal strip starting on the lateral side of the midfoot anchor, running around the heel and finishing on the medial aspect of the anchor (Fig 1.5b)
- Continue to apply vertical and horizontal strips until support is adequate. Each strip should overlap the previous strip by a third (Fig 1.5c)
- Apply locking strips in the same fashion as the anchor strips

Double heel lock

Aim: to control calcaneal movement following an inversion ankle sprain. Can be applied in conjunction with the basket weave tape above.

Tape: 3.8 cm adhesive zinc oxide tape.

Application:
- Starting on the medial aspect of the shin, angle the tape down posterior to the lateral malleolus, over the Achilles tendon to the postero-medial calcaneus
- Draw the tape firmly from the medial to the lateral aspect of the calcaneus into eversion (Fig 1.6a)
- Continue up over the dorsum of the foot to the medial malleolus and laterally around the Achilles tendon (Fig 1.6b)
- Continue inferiorly down posterior to the lateral malleolus, medially under the heel and pull up on the medial aspect of the ankle at the level of the navicular (Fig 1.6c)
- Continue high over the dorsum of the foot, finishing laterally high above the level of the lateral malleolus (Fig 1.6d)

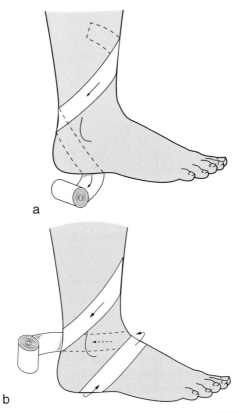

a

b

Fig 1.6 Double heel lock to control calcaneal motion: (a) Step 1 – around the heel medial to lateral, (b) Step 2 – over the dorsum of the foot,

(Continued)

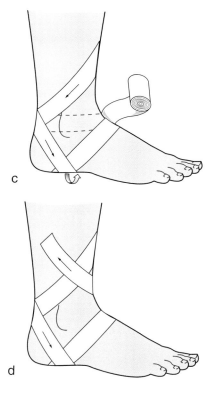

c

d

Fig 1.6—cont'd (c) Step 3 – around the heel lateral to medial and (d) Step 4 – completed tape.

Know your first aid

Injuries in a sporting arena are always a cause for concern and can sometimes cause panic. To keep a clear and level head during an incident and manage any scenario most effectively, it is essential to follow a logical sequence of actions. If you follow the same process for even the most minor injuries, you will have a greater ability to deal with a medical emergency. These principles are discussed in detail here and laid out in a Serious Injury Algorithm in Fig 1.7.

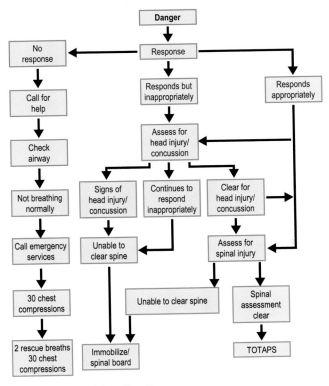

Fig 1.7 Serious Injury Algorithm.

It is essential that all clinicians maintain their competency in this area, and update their knowledge and skills by completing regular **recognized** training courses. Many governing bodies such as the Rugby Football Union (RFU) will only recognize certain training courses as meeting an appropriate standard. Anyone looking to update their first aid and injury management skills should find out whether a course meets these requirements. The Association of Chartered Physiotherapists in Sports Medicine (ACPSM) has different requirements for different levels of accreditation.

Step 1: danger

Your immediate priority is to assess the area for danger – to yourself, the injured athlete and others in the vicinity. Ensure that it is safe for you to enter the area and then warn others caring for the athlete against any unnecessary movements in case a spinal injury has occurred.

Step 2: response

If the athlete does not respond to you spontaneously, you need to try to get a response by holding their shoulders and asking them to open their eyes. If you get no response, you should follow the ABC principles of resuscitation.

Step 3: airway, breathing and circulation (ABC)

Guidelines for resuscitation undergo constant review. At the time of writing in 2010, the Resuscitation Council (UK) has just published updated guidelines.

All clinicians should refer regularly to the Resuscitation Council (UK) website (www.resus.org.uk) for the latest recommendations regarding management. The Serious Injury Algorithm incorporates the guidelines published in 2005.

Airway

Look for the following:

- Is the athlete agitated or cyanosed?
- Is there excessive accessory muscle use?
- Are there any facial injuries or evidence of trauma to the neck or trachea?
- Are there any teeth missing?
- Is there bleeding from the mouth or nose?
- Has the athlete vomited?
- Listen for abnormal breathing sounds – gurgling/stridor/hoarseness
- **Do not roll the athlete** unless there is bleeding from the mouth or nose or vomiting.
- To open the airway – use a chin lift or jaw thrust manoeuvre.
- If you suspect the athlete may have sustained a spinal injury, pull the jaw forward to open the airway rather than tilting the head backwards.
- **Do not insert your finger into the athlete's mouth** to clear the airway. If you have access to a rigid suction device, this can be used.
- If the athlete is breathing but remains unresponsive, consider inserting either an oropharyngeal or nasopharyngeal airway to assist airway management.
- **Remember – airway maintenance always takes precedence over a potential spinal injury.**

Breathing and circulation

Follow the Resuscitation Council (UK) guidelines.

Step 4: assessment for head injury/ concussion

In ascertaining if the athlete is conscious and responding appropriately, dangerous movements of the athlete's head and neck may occur as they turn to look at you and respond to your questions. Taking hold of the athlete's head and instructing them not to move while you ascertain the extent of their injuries will stop this. Do not move the player unless this is necessary for saftey. This includes lying them down if they are standing up. If they are standing, perform your assessment in this position.

Introduce yourself with your name and profession if you are unknown to the athlete or player.

Screen for a head injury or concussion by questioning the patient about the following:

- Headache
- Blurred vision
- Nausea
- Dizziness

Follow this by examining the patient for signs of confusion, agitation, memory loss or inappropriate responses to simple questions.

To rule out a head injury/concussion the athlete must be able to respond appropriately to simple questions:

- What is your name?
- Who are we playing?
- Which quarter/half are we in?
- Who is winning?
- What is the score?
- What position are you playing?

Concussion should be suspected if the player has experienced a loss of consciousness or demonstrates an altered mental state or inappropriate responses to questioning.

All players with a suspected head injury and concussion should be referred for an urgent medical review.

Monitoring concussion

If a player is suffering from concussion or a minor head injury, it is essential that they are monitored for signs of a deteriorating condition until they have fully recovered.

Possible signs and symptoms include:
- Confusion or irritability
- Drowsiness/unconsciousness
- Severe or progressive headaches

- Blurred vision/dizziness
- Repeated vomiting
- Slurred speech

This information is provided to friends and relatives by A&E departments; however, it may be that they are not present to receive this information. If this is the case, you must ensure that the information is given in both verbal and written form to the person caring for the individual.

The player must not be left alone. If you are travelling away, good practice is for a member of the medical team to remain with the player, including spending the night with them monitoring symptoms and signs while the player remains awake. Remember – it is not possible to assess for deterioration if the player is asleep!

If the player is unable to answer questions coherently and appropriately, you cannot rule out the presence of a spinal injury.

If the presence of a spinal injury cannot be ruled out, it must be assumed that the player has a spinal injury. They must be treated as if they have a spinal injury, until it is ruled out by medical investigations.

A SPINAL INJURY MUST BE ASSUMED UNTIL IT CAN BE EXCLUDED.

Once you have determined that the player does not have a head injury/concussion, you should screen for the presence of a spinal injury.

To screen for a potential spinal injury, you need to question the player about:

- Presence of spinal pain or significant stiffness
- Central/midline tenderness
- Presence of any pins and needles or absence of sensation
- Feeling of altered power/tone

You also need to examine the patient for:

- Tenderness over the spinal vertebrae
- Obvious spinal deformity/step
- Significant spasm

If all of these elements are clear, the spine can be considered stable and the patient is permitted to move their neck. At this stage, you should ask about pain, pins and needles, numbness and weakness, as a missed injury may become apparent with movement.

The player should be instructed to turn their head from side to side and to look up and down. This should be done both in the position in which the player is first assessed (often lying down) and also while standing.

Management of a suspected spinal injury

If you suspect a spinal injury has occurred or you are unable to clear the spine because of a lack of an appropriate response from the player, you must immobilize the head and neck in the position in which you find the athlete. The aim of first aid in this situation is not to move them from that position and one person must be specifically designated to maintain the head and neck position.

Do not move the athlete's head into the midline.

A rigid cervical collar can be used only if the athlete's cervical spine is in the midline. If you find the athlete in any other position, their head and neck must be maintained in this position by the designated individual until further medical help arrives.

If it becomes necessary to roll the athlete with a suspected spinal injury because they are vomiting or bleeding from the mouth, log rolling must be used.

Log rolling requires at least 4 people who know the procedure to ensure that the manoeuvre maintains spinal alignment. It is also the technique used to roll an injured player onto a spinal board.

Using a spinal board

Even if a spinal board is available at a competition, it should only ever be used when individuals are familiar and confident in moving a player with a suspected spinal injury.

The required competency elements include:

• Application of a rigid collar (see above regarding application)

- Log rolling
- Application of straps and head blocks to the spinal board
- Carrying the player and spinal board from the field of play

Moving an injured athlete

An injured athlete should be moved from the field or arena only if airway, breathing and circulation (ABC) are all stable and either the spine has been deemed stable or the athlete is immobilized in a rigid collar on a spinal board.

If this is impossible, the athlete must not be moved under any circumstances until medical help is available, except for potential danger to the athlete or clinician. This may mean abandoning a game or competition or moving to an alternative field or venue.

 Practice and confidence are the key to managing any serious incident. Medical teams should set aside regular sessions to practise On Field Management so that each team member is familiar with their role. For individuals, regular updates and practice sessions are recommended.

TOTAPS

For any non-serious injury (strain/sprain), TOTAPS (Table 1.2) is a relatively safe and effective injury diagnosis process for pitchside management.

If you elect to remove a player from the field:

- Keep them warm
- Decide whether urgent hospital referral is required
- Monitor for shock
- Monitor mental state

Table 1.2 TOTAPS – pitchside diagnostic process

Action	
Talk to the injured player	If you did not witness the injury can the player describe what happened? Did you hear any unusual sounds? Where is the injury? What is the pain like? Any pins and needles? Is there any obvious deformity?
Observe (compare to uninjured side)	Mental state/consciousness Swelling Deformity Bleeding/bruising Spontaneous movement
Touch	Tenderness – observe level of distress Swelling Heat Deformity
Active movement	Available range Associated pain Functional movement of the limb
Passive movement	Available range Pain response Laxity or instability Guarding/splinting
Skill test	Sport-specific movements – walking – hopping/running – throwing/catching – weight-bearing for upper limb **Determine ability to continue playing**

When to call for an ambulance

- Head injury
- Suspected spinal injury
- Deteriorating patient
- The athlete has suffered thoracic trauma and is having difficulty breathing
- Compound or serious fracture – alteration to peripheral pulses
- The athlete has vomited blood (suspect significant internal injury)
- The athlete is in shock

Know when to refer to hospital

This is always going to be a judgment call, but some useful guidelines include:

- Head injury and/or significant concussion
- Significant neck or back pain in which a neurological injury has been ruled out
- Chest or abdominal trauma without breathing difficulties or vomiting
- Other fractures
- Serious trauma – flail chest, dislocations with suspected bony involvement
- Dislocations of the thumb or index finger (do not reduce yourself)
- Large lacerations or open wounds
- DOUBT!

 Never let a player go to hospital alone. Ensure there is a designated individual to go with them who is fully briefed (ideally with some written documentation from you) on the player's condition. Ensure you take a contact number from them so you can gain an update on the player's status.

It should never become necessary for you to leave other players unsupported to escort someone to hospital. If no-one else is available, the coach should go with the player. If it is necessary to leave the playing arena and follow a player to hospital, inform all coaching and management staff as well as any opposition medical personnel. Remember to take cash and/or a credit card with you for food or transportation. Also ensure you take something warm to put on. It is not unusual for medical staff to go into shock after dealing with a serious incident. Call from the hospital once the player is stable or under medical care to inform the coaching staff of the player's condition.

Know what to document

In the event of any injury, thorough and accurate recording is required. A simple, standardized form makes this easy and ensures all the relevant information is recorded.

Check the requirements of any organization you are working with and use their standard form.

If a standard form is not available, it is a good idea to create your own and use it regularly.

Form 1.2 is an example form based on that of Sports Medicine Australia illustrating the information that should be recorded.

Form 1.2   Injury report form

Player's name: . . . .   Gender: . . . .

Contact details: . . . .

Date: . . . .   Time: . . . .

Venue: . . . .   Team: . . . .

Clinician's name: . . . .

Serious injury assessment:
Airway: . . . .

Breathing: . . . .

Circulation: . . . .

Concussion: . . . .

Spine: . . . .

Reason for   HPC:
presentation:
  • New injury
  • Aggravation
  • Recurrent

- Illness
- Other
- Body part:

TOTAPS:

T

O

T

A

P

S

Cause of injury:

- ❑ Hit by the ball
- ❑ Collision with another player (own team/opposition)
- ❑ Collision with stationary object

- ❑ Slip/trip/stumble/fall
- ❑ Overuse
- ❑ Overexertion
- ❑ Landing
- ❑ Hydration related
- ❑ Temperature related
- ❑ Other

Suspected nature of injury/illness:

- ❑ Soft tissue
- ❑ Dislocation
- ❑ Bony
- ❑ Wound/abrasion
- ❑ Internal
- ❑ Illness
- ❑ Other medical
- ❑ Other

Initial management:

- ❑ None given
- ❑ Advice only
- ❑ RICE (Rest, Ice, Compression, Elevation) + warnings and advice

- ❑ Strapping
- ❑ Sling/splint
- ❑ Wound care
- ❑ Asthma
- ❑ Hypo/hyperthermia
- ❑ CPR
- ❑ Referred
- ❑ Rest/monitor
- ❑ Other

Referral

- ❑ GP
- ❑ Ambulance
- ❑ Hospital
- ❑ Other

Injured player told that if injury/illness does NOT improve in the following 24 hours they MUST seek further advice from their own medical professional

- ❑ YES

Player's signature:
Advice given:

- ❑ Cleared to continue playing
- ❑ Return to play with restrictions
- ❑ Unable to return at present
- ❑ Requires clearance prior to playing

Clinician's signature:　　　**Qualifications:**　　　**Date:**

From Sports Medicine Australia.

Know when to refer on

Clinicians working with large professional teams are usually fortunate enough to be part of a multidisciplinary medical group in which joint consultations for players are common. This has many advantages. All clinicians bring different skills and experiences to the consultation, ensuring multiple diagnoses and contributing factors are considered when reviewing players. Experience plays a large role in developing clinical skills. Working with experienced clinicians provides less experienced members of the team with the opportunity to learn pattern recognition of less common conditions as well as management strategies for these and conditions encountered more commonly.

If you are working on your own, it is important to know when you should seek a second opinion or an onward referral for a condition.

These include:

- Athletes for whom you are not sure of the diagnosis
- Athletes who are not responding to treatment as expected based upon your diagnosis
- Athletes whose condition is deteriorating
- Athletes who are in significant levels of pain – not sleeping, requiring ongoing medication use
- Athletes who are experiencing recurrent episodes of the same or similar conditions
- Athletes who are underperforming for unknown reasons (not musculoskeletal). An athlete in this scenario may be suffering from overtraining or underperformance syndrome, which requires medical intervention by a clinician specializing in this field. Alternatively, there may be a serious underlying pathology of a systemic nature.

Know when to arrange further investigations

As MRI becomes increasingly more affordable and available, it can be tempting to request a scan for anything for which the diagnosis is unclear or is not responding to treatment. However, just because an MRI gives you a 3D representation of both the bony and soft tissue structures, this does not mean it is always the best scan to request, as it does not always give the clearest indication of the suspected injury. It is my experience that providing as much clinical information as possible, including a differential diagnosis, will allow the radiology department to determine the most appropriate scan for the suspected condition.

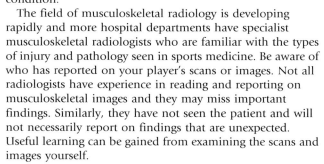

The field of musculoskeletal radiology is developing rapidly and more hospital departments have specialist musculoskeletal radiologists who are familiar with the types of injury and pathology seen in sports medicine. Be aware of who has reported on your player's scans or images. Not all radiologists have experience in reading and reporting on musculoskeletal images and they may miss important findings. Similarly, they have not seen the patient and will not necessarily report on findings that are unexpected. Useful learning can be gained from examining the scans and images yourself.

Assessment and diagnosis of the injured athlete

Introduction

The purpose of this pocketbook is not to be a definitive text on musculoskeletal examination; there are plenty of other texts that deliver this very well. Instead we present the fundamental principles that apply to both the subjective history and objective examination for most peripheral joints and a basic screen for spinal examination. Also included are special questions and tests for specific anatomical areas and injuries. Any of these examinations should detect the majority of common injuries in both the acute and chronic presentations, but they will not pick up every single pathology. The fundamental principles will be covered in this section and special questions and tests will be covered in the injury-specific sections.

We use a novel approach to the injury-specific sections. Clinical reasoning in patient management requires the clinician to generate a number of possible diagnostic hypotheses which are then "tested" using the patient's responses to both subjective questioning and physical examination. Through interaction with clinicians, the authors have recognized that identifying diagnostic hypotheses is often difficult. The injury-specific section describes several diagnostic possibilities for each region, against which the clinician can test and compare their patient's presentation. Whilst we all know that two individuals presenting with the same condition will rarely present with exactly the same features, familiar patterns present both in the history and examination. Some of these patterns are more common than others and we have used our years of clinical and teaching experience in an attempt to allocate how frequently these occur in order to assist typical pattern recognition of these injuries. We employ the following tick system to give a rough idea how frequently these signs and symptoms present:

Patterns of positive findings

✓✓✓	Nearly always
✓✓	Often
✓	Sometimes

Two other issues to bear in mind when you are using the injury-specific sections:

1. The degree of injury. This could be mild–severe, Grade 1–Grade 3; however you want to classify it. Unless it is indicated otherwise (e.g. rupture of the Achilles tendon) we have accounted for injuries in the middle of the injury spectrum.

2. The timing of your examination. In the acute phase, if you are pitchside and get to examine the athlete straight away, you are more likely to get positive tests where positive tests exist. Examination of the same athlete in the clinic 24–48 hours later may not elicit the same positive signs if sufficient pain and swelling has developed. In this situation it might not be possible to complete a full examination until the acute stage has settled. In the chronic stage this may be not so much of an issue.

Examination of peripheral joints

Subjective history

Caveat – any athlete training and competing on a regular basis who presents with symptoms will naturally try and relate these to their sporting activity, when in fact the two may not be associated. It is important to establish the exact activity, cause and time of onset – if the athlete is unable to do this there must be an index of suspicion that this may not be a "traumatic" musculoskeletal injury.

2

Assessment and diagnosis of the injured athlete

Taking a good subjective history is a skill that needs to be developed – try and ask open questions and avoid any leading questions. If at the first time of asking you do not have all the information you were seeking, try and paraphrase the question without giving too much information. For example, "can you tell me what your problem is?" i.e. do not presume it is pain that is the problem here – you want to hear the description of their problem in their own words without any autosuggestion of what they should be experiencing or telling you.

A detailed history is important to establish what you are dealing with and you need to determine the following:

1. Differentiate whether you are dealing with an acute or chronic injury.
2. Is it a traumatic or overuse injury?
3. Establish the mechanism – was it a contact or non-contact injury?
4. Did any swelling occur? Where, how quickly and how long did it take to resolve?
5. What are the problems now?

- Location of symptoms – localized or vague? Can they put their finger on it or do they generally rub an area with the palm of their hand? This may be important to differentiate localized or referred pain
- Nature of symptoms. Pain – sharp, dull/ache; deep/superficial?
- Severity? A patient specific activity VAS scale out of 10 (Form 2.1)
- Behaviour of symptoms — intermittent or continuous? Need to differentiate between mechanical and chemical pain. In the acute inflammatory stage where a chemical response is underway there may well be continuous pain. In the absence of an acute injury, continual pain is not normal and is indicative of:
  - Serious pathology
  - Psychosocial factors

Form 2.1   Patient-Specific Functional Scale

This useful questionnaire can be used to quantify activity limitation and measure functional outcomes for patients with any orthopaedic condition

Initial assessment:
I am going to ask you to identify up to three important activities that you are unable to do or are having difficulty with as a result of your _____ problem. Today, are there any activities that you are unable to do or having difficulty with because of your _____ problem? (Clinician: show scale to patient and have the patient rate each activity.)

Follow-up assessments:
When I assessed you on (state previous assessment date), you told me that you had difficulty with (read all activities from list at a time). Today, do you still have difficulty with: (read and have patient score each item in the list)?

Patient specific activity scoring scheme (point to one number):

0	1	2	3	4	5	6	7	8	9	10

Unable to
perform
activity

Able to perform
activity at the
same level as
before injury or
problem

(Date and Score)

Activity	Initial					
1.						
2.						
3.						
4.						
5.						
Additional						
Additional						

Total score = sum of the activity scores/number of activities
Minimum detectable change (90% CI) for average score = 2 points
Minimum detectable change (90% CI) for single activity score = 3 points

PSFS developed by: Stratford P, Gill C, Westaway M and Binkley J (1995) Assessing disability and change on individual patients: a report of a patient specific measure. Physiotherapy Canada 47:258-263.
Reproduced with the permission of the authors.

- Do the symptoms occur on a daily basis? Try and establish if there is any pattern
- Red flags – check for night pain

6. Irritability – how easily are the symptoms provoked and how quickly once provoked do these settle down? If the irritability is high, this might guide your choice and order of examination techniques. Establish the aggravating and easing factors – the mechanics of these may help indicate what the problem is and also how to manage it. An example of highly irritable back pain may take 5 minutes of sitting to flare it up and then they may have to lie flat for 2 hours for it to settle. Compare this with an example of knee pain that takes all day walking around to come on and will then ease off after sitting down for 5 minutes
7. Family history
8. Medication history
9. Social history

At the end of the subjective examination an experienced clinician should be approximately 80% certain of what they are dealing with and will tailor the physical examination accordingly to prove and/or disprove this working hypothesis.

Physical examination

For peripheral joints, the contralateral limb should be used for comparison as long as there are no problems with the other side. Always assess the contralateral limb first so the athlete knows what you are about to do and what it should feel like **before** testing the injured side.

From the subjective examination you should know the nature, severity and irritability of the condition and what tests are likely to provoke any symptoms. The order of the examination may need to be modified to take this into account. **Observation** Biomechanical evaluation in standing and walking (Table 2.1). Check for swelling and temperature changes if necessary.

Table 2.1 Biomechanical Evaluation

1. What you need to do?
2. What do your findings mean in relation to the presentation? Picking out biomechanical anomalies is easy – most people have them. The KEY feature is linking these to the athletes sign and symptoms (see example in patellofemoral knee pain, page 84).
3. Can you change the signs and symptoms by altering the biomechanics?

Part 1: Static Evaluation

In weight-bearing:

Pelvis: In anterior or posterior tilt? If yes, are there any compensatory changes?

Hip: Femoral anteversion: Craig test

Knee: Varus/valgus/hyperextended

Foot: Position: Forefoot pronation or supination; Rearfoot calcaneal eversion

Part 2: Dynamic Evaluation

Gait

Small knee bend

Single leg stance   Increases demand and requires more control

Lunge

Step-up and Step-down

Observation during task: (i) change in spinal position (ii) pelvic position (iii) hip abd/add/rotation (iv) dynamic knee valgus (v) patella position relative to the femur (vi) foot position

Note: Analysis of running should ideally be done on a treadmill with a video camera.

Active ROM It is obviously important to see how much movement there is, but perhaps more crucial is to see how willing the athlete is to move the limb, the quality of the movement and to then note the onset of any pain.

Passive ROM The joint or muscle being tested should be taken to end of range and overpressure applied. The examiner evaluates the range of movement, when resistance occurs during range, the end feel and presence of any pain reported.

Resisted muscle test The muscle to be tested should be put into mid-range and tested isometrically in the first instance. The examiner should try and ensure that minimal movement occurs during the test and the muscle is tested maximally.

The examiner is evaluating for the presence of pain and/or weakness.

Ligament tests The basic principle for ligament testing is that the examiner should know the anatomy of the ligament to be tested. The joint should be placed in the optimal position to test the ligament and then taken to the end of range to "wind" the ligament up, and overpressure applied. The examiner is evaluating for the presence of laxity and/or pain. The most common ligament injuries are covered in the injury-specific section.

Special tests These will include anything that does not strictly fit into the other categories.

Functional tests These should be specific to the presentation and structure being tested. For example, if an athlete presents with anterior knee pain which comes on after running for a mile and little is found on examination, then you may need to send them out to run for a mile and then reassess them. Functional tests should be selected for sport specificity and the stage of the pathology. Additionally, these can be quite provocative, e.g. triple leg cross-over hop (see Fig 4.3), and therefore should be introduced incrementally starting with lower demand tests and progressing appropriately.

At the end of examination you should have established a working diagnosis and a management plan which may consist of further investigation and conservative or surgical management.

Common Injuries in the Upper limb

Shoulder

Acute shoulder injuries

Glenohumeral dislocation

The shoulder is the most commonly dislocated joint. Shoulder dislocation is one of the most common traumatic injuries in sport and occurs frequently in contact sports such as rugby or judo. It can occur in a posterior or inferior direction, but 95% of dislocations occur anteriorly.

Subjective:

Anterior dislocation occurs when the arm is positioned in abduction and external rotation – may be associated with external force from an opponent or a fall ✓✓✓

Immediate, severe pain associated with the injury. The athlete describes a sensation of the shoulder "popping out" ✓✓ ✓

Unable to play on ✓✓✓

Pins and needles, numbness or discoloration through the arm to the hand in the presence of damage to nerve or blood vessels ✓✓

Subsequent feeling of instability or episodes of giving way in the absence of pain ✓✓✓

Objective:

Obvious deformity – head of humerus sitting anteriorly – normal shoulder contours lost ✓✓✓

Active and passive movement – limited by pain and severe muscle spasm ✓✓✓

Patient holds shoulder supported close to the body and resists movements, especially into abduction/external rotation ✓✓

Positive apprehension sign ✓✓✓ (Fig 2.1). This testing is only undertaken in an athlete with chronic symptoms. In acute cases, pain and muscle spasm will prevent the therapist from being able to position the shoulder for testing

Associated injury:

Bankart lesion – tear of the glenoid labrum
Bony Bankart – glenoid fracture associated with labral tear
Hills–Sachs lesion–cortical depression in the head of the humerus as a result of impaction of the humeral head against the anterior inferior glenoid rim

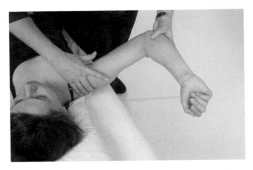

Fig 2.1 Apprehension test for anterior shoulder instability.

The presence of any of these associated injuries increases the likelihood of recurrent dislocations

Management: (see also Case Study in Section 3 p 213)

DO NOT ATTEMPT TO REDUCE THE DISLOCATION ON FIELD

Immediate management – sling support/pain relief/medical attention to relocate the joint

Immobilization – external rotation vs. internal rotation Some research suggests that shoulders immobilized in external rotation, as opposed to the more conventional position of internal rotation with the arm across the body, may be less likely to experience repeat dislocations. In external rotation, the glenohumeral ligament and labrum are brought into a more normal anatomical position and are therefore more likely to heal in this proper position. Practically, immobilization in external rotation can make daily function quite difficult and this form of immobilization is still quite uncommon. Patients also need to be put into this position of immobilization within 3 days of the dislocation for it to be at all effective

Athletes are initially managed with a conservative rehabilitation programme aimed at improving rotator cuff and shoulder strength and control. The clinician should have a limited tolerance/low threshold for surgical review in elite athletes or people playing contact sports if conservative management does not reduce sensations of instability and apprehension

Presence of instability 3 months after injury would suggest a need for surgical intervention to prevent recurrent dislocations in active individuals

Older athletes, with stiffer shoulders, are less likely to have recurrent symptoms and may manage with a conservative approach

Acromioclavicular joint sprain

Acromioclavicular (AC) joint strains are thought to account for about 40% of all shoulder injuries and almost always occur as a result of either a fall onto the shoulder or the outstretched hand (cycling, judo, horse riding) or a direct blow to the shoulder (contact sports) ✓✓✓

Subjective:

Significant, superficial pain localized to the region of the AC joint ✓✓✓

Difficulty with elevation movements above 60° – degree of limitation dependent upon the severity of the injury ✓✓

Difficulty sleeping on the affected shoulder ✓✓✓

Objective:

Pain and swelling directly over the AC joint ✓✓✓

Step deformity – between the clavicle and acromion ✓

Active movement – limited by pain ✓✓

Full range of passive glenohumeral motion ✓✓✓

Specific tenderness on palpation of AC joint ✓✓✓

Investigations:

An X-ray may be ordered to rule out a fracture and determine the extent of the joint separation

Management:

Immediate management – sling support and pain relief – PRICE (Protection, Rest, Ice, Compression, Elevation) Physiotherapy is often not necessary in the case of mild sprains, but may be required in the case of higher grades of injury or in cases where the athlete is slow to regain range of motion and function. In these instances, manual therapy will be required to regain shoulder mobility, with appropriate strength and control exercises used concurrently In very rare cases surgery may be required

Rotator cuff tear

Most rotator cuff tears occur as a result of overuse and tend to occur in people over the age of 40 ✓✓✓
Acute tears of the cuff are the result of trauma and may occur in association with other injuries or excessively forceful activation of the muscle group in a long lever situation (gymnastics/kayaking)

Subjective:

Sudden onset of pain over the region of the deltoid insertion (referred pain) ✓✓✓

Pain settles reasonably quickly within a few days ✓✓

"Popping" sensation in the shoulder associated with the injury ✓

Immediate onset of weakness associated with shoulder elevation—dependent upon the severity of the injury ✓✓

Objective:

Painful and limited shoulder elevation (flexion and abduction) ✓✓

Poor movement pattern of elevation with excessive scapular motion to compensate for inefficient glenohumeral motion ✓✓✓

Non-specific tenderness on palpation over the region of the rotator cuff – often difficult to localize tear ✓✓

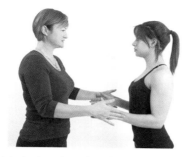

Fig 2.2 Resisted external rotation of the shoulder: infraspinatus and teres minor.

Specific tests:

Muscle strength tests for the isolated muscle will indicate which element of the cuff is torn
NB: In the acute stage all tests may be pain inhibited

- External rotation – infraspinatus and teres minor (Fig 2.2)
- Internal rotation – subscapularis (Fig 2.3)
- Empty can test – supraspinatus

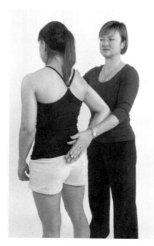

Fig 2.3 Resisted internal rotation of the shoulder: subscapularis.

2

Assessment and diagnosis of the injured athlete

Management:

PRICE

Passive/assisted active range of motion exercises – to maintain mobility and avoid shoulder stiffness

Graduated strengthening exercises targeting the rotator cuff

Chronic shoulder injuries

Shoulder impingement

This is a very general term that describes the etiological process, in which an element of the rotator cuff musculature is "impinged" between the humeral head and the acromion during elevation activities. It is therefore common in athletes involved in repetitive overhead activities. Shoulder impingement is usually described as either primary, where the cause of the impingement is a structural anomaly of the shoulder or secondary, where the impingement occurs because of poor motor control around the shoulder. In this way, an overlap between secondary shoulder impingement and instability exists and the two often occur concurrently ✓✓

Examples of primary causes include an altered acromial shape or bony spurs as a result of degenerative changes.

Subjective:

Minor pain in the shoulder region at rest, increased significantly with elevation movements ✓✓✓

Pain localized to the anterior/ lateral shoulder only extending as far as the deltoid insertion and not into the trapezius region ✓✓✓

Pain and restriction with hand behind back movements ✓✓

Difficulty lying on the affected shoulder at night ✓

Objective:

Patient's symptoms reproduced with active flexion and abduction – arc of pain from 80° to 120° ✓✓✓

Full passive range of motion ✓✓✓
Motion restricted primarily by pain rather than stiffness ✓✓✓
Active movements which are painful can be performed
painfree passively ✓✓
Minor strength deficits ✓
NB: Suspect a cuff tear in any case with significant weakness

Investigations:

In cases of primary impingement, an X-ray (outlet view) is
useful in determining whether degenerative changes exist in
the AC joint that may be contributing to the impingement

Special tests:

There are several tests for impingement (Neer, Hawkins–
Kennedy) and all are designed to reproduce the compression
of the rotator cuff between the bony elements (Fig 2.4)
Copeland's test (an extension of Neer's test) – abduction in
the scapula plane with the shoulder in internal rotation
causes mid-arc pain which is abolished with abduction in
external rotation ✓✓✓

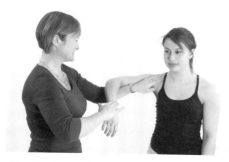

Fig 2.4 Hawkins–Kennedy test for shoulder impingement.

2

Assessment and diagnosis of the injured athlete

Neer's test, in which an athlete's impingement pain is abolished on administration of a subacromial injection of local anaesthetic, can be useful in confirming the source of pain, but will not help direct treatment

Associated injury:

Secondary impingement is defined as rotator cuff impingement that occurs secondary to a functional decrease in the supraspinatus outlet space due to underlying instability/poor motor control of the glenohumeral joint. It is a more common cause than the presence of degenerative changes in young athletes, and should always form part of the examination process

Ongoing impingement may result in:

- Microtrauma to the tendon and inflammatory changes
- Bursitis
- Calcific tendonitis

In older athletes, rotator cuff tears may result from ongoing impingement

Management: (see also Case Study in Section 3 p 222)

Correction of motor control deficits – scapular or glenohumeral joint

- rotator cuff rotational control
- scapular control – prevent excessive protraction and downward rotation (Fig 2.5)

NB: Restricted motion may also contribute to motor control changes – need to examine glenohumeral (Fig 2.6) and scapular mobility passively

Soft tissue techniques:

Subacromial injection often useful to provide "window of opportunity" for rehabilitation to be effective. Settles inflammatory response

Surgery usually indicated in cases of primary impingement

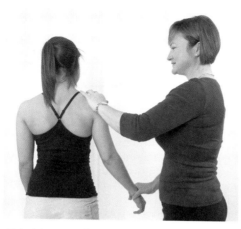

Fig 2.5 Retraining scapular upward rotation.

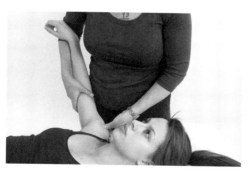

Fig 2.6 Glenohumeral abduction with longitudinal glide (manual therapy).

Shoulder instability

Shoulder instability is a common sporting problem with multiple manifestations that can make its management complex. Numerous classification systems exist. The Stanmore classification is useful in recognizing the spectrum of presentations (Fig 2.7).

This suggests that there are three broad reasons why shoulders present with symptoms of instability. Firstly, a structural problem exists, either because the capsuloligamentous structures have become deficient as a result of major injury (traumatic structural), or secondly, already slightly compromised structures have been subjected to repetitive microtrauma that has led to a loss of stability (atraumatic structural). The third broad reason is an alteration in muscle recruitment around the shoulder

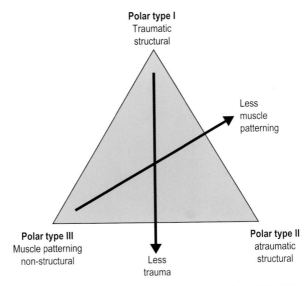

Fig 2.7 The Stanmore Classification of shoulder instability. With permission from www.shoulderdoc.co.uk.

complex (scapulothoracic/glenohumeral) causing a loss of the ideal orientation of the glenoid and humeral head in relation to each other during movement (muscle patterning).

Degrees of overlap of pathology and therefore signs and symptoms exist that require careful history-taking and examination to determine the presence or absence of each component.

The three broad categories will be discussed below

Subjective:

Traumatic structural

Significant trauma ✓✓✓

Unilateral symptoms ✓✓✓

Dislocating position – abduction/external rotation – anterior ✓✓✓

Unable to self relocate

Atraumatic structural

Common in throwers and swimmers where shoulder is subjected to overload/fatigue – develop microtrauma

Recurrent ✓✓

Minor activity – associated with sensation that shoulder has "popped out" ✓✓✓

Patient reports certain positions that result in dislocation/subluxation ✓✓✓

Bilateral ✓✓

Self relocate/require minimal assistance ✓✓✓

Muscle patterning

Recurrent ✓✓

Bilateral ✓✓

Able to "dislocate" voluntarily – "party trick" ✓✓

Painless dislocation ✓✓✓

Self relocate/require minimal assistance ✓✓✓

Objective:

Traumatic structural

Significant muscle spasm
Positive test for ligamentous laxity following relocation ✓✓✓
(Figs 2.1 and 2.8)

Atraumatic structural

Positive test for ligamentous laxity ✓✓✓
Evidence of overload/fatigue of shoulder stabilizing muscles ✓

Muscle patterning

Ligamentous laxity testing NAD ✓✓✓
Able to "dislocate" voluntarily – "party trick" ✓✓
Abnormal pattern of shoulder control – scapulo-
humeral ✓✓✓

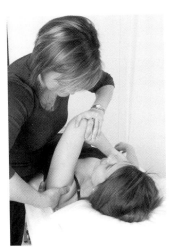

Fig 2.8 Testing the integrity of the posterior shoulder structures.

Management:

PRICE

Multidisiplinary team approach essential

Traumatic structural

Reduction of dislocation in A&E

Sling – 2/3 weeks ± painkillers/NSAIDS

± physiotherapy rehabilitation – ROM and strength

Emphasis on proprioceptive re-education

Severe/recurrent – Repair of Bankart lesion

Atraumatic structural

Rehabilitation – motor control

Proprioceptive retraining

Address areas of soft tissue/joint restriction – commonly posterior capsule

Muscle patterning

Rehabilitation aimed at addressing the sequencing pattern of muscle activation – commonly the large muscles of the glenohumeral joint – latissimus dorsi/pectoralis major/ deltoids are overactive

Soft tissue work

Address control of glenohumeral joint movement with rotator cuff control

Need to review entire kinetic chain – often poor posture generally – trunk control

Rotator cuff tear

Athletes with chronic cuff damage are usually over the age of 40 ✓✓✓. They often complain of a history of minor shoulder pain and irritation that worsens suddenly as the result of a minor incident or period of excessive activity in which the arm is raised above shoulder height.

2

Assessment and diagnosis of the injured athlete

Subjective:

Affected shoulder is the dominant arm ✓✓✓

Pain has gradually got worse over time – difficult to localize – most specific in the region of the deltoid ✓✓✓

Restriction to shoulder function due to pain and weakness ✓✓✓

Night pain – unable to lie on affected shoulder ✓✓✓

Objective:

Painful limitation of elevation movement with associated weakness ✓✓✓

Poor movement pattern of elevation with excessive scapular motion to compensate for inefficient glenohumeral motion ✓✓✓

Other movements affected by long-standing changes in cuff function and control ✓✓✓

Non-specific tenderness on palpation over the region of the rotator cuff – often difficult to localize tear ✓✓

Weakness evident on testing of specific cuff muscles
NB: May be difficult to isolate one muscle group as all may be weak and/or painful on testing ✓✓
(see Figs 2.2 and 2.3)

Management:

Pain control – may benefit from local injection therapy (local anaesthesia and corticosteroid) to reduce inflammatory changes and pain inhibition in order to provide a window of opportunity for rehabilitation

Graduated cuff control exercises – focus on rotation and control with elevation movements

Specific scapular re-education is necessary if shoulder dysfunction has been present for some time

Surgery may be required if conservative management has failed (large tears) or if the patient has high demands from the shoulder for work or sporting activities

C5 shoulder syndrome

The C5–6 vertebral motion segment is the level most commonly involved in the development of neck and upper limb symptoms. This is probably due to gravitational effects and altered postural alignment. Clinicians treating athletes with upper limb pain often fail to examine the cervical spine adequately, especially when the athlete's symptoms are reproduced with movements of the arm.

Subjective:

Pain in the shoulder and upper arm region ✓✓✓

Dull, aching quality of pain – mimics pain from the somatic structures of the shoulder ✓✓✓

Symptoms aggravated by movements of the arm and shoulder, especially elevation above 90° ✓✓✓

No reported neck pain or other symptoms ✓✓

Objective:

Active cervical movement tests all NAD including overpressure ✓✓✓

Neurological assessment NAD

Hypomobile and tenderness present on manual segmental examination of C5–6 vertebral level – unilateral and comparable with the side of symptoms ✓✓✓

Positive upper limb neural provocation test – commonly ULNPT 1 ✓ (Fig 2.9)

Management:

Manual therapy – mobilization ± manipulation directed to C5–6 level

Correction of upper quadrant movement dysfunctions – important to examine the relationship between spinal movement and upper limb movement and control. Address cervical control, scapular control and rotator cuff function

2

Assessment and diagnosis of the injured athlete

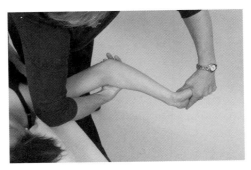

Fig 2.9 Upper limb neural provocation test 1.

Elbow

Lateral elbow pain

Lateral elbow pain is commonly referred to as "tennis elbow", but this entity is certainly not restricted to tennis players. It is also known as "lateral epicondylitis", but given the current understanding of the underlying pathology, the term "tendinosis" would be more appropriate.

Subjective:

Acute or insidious onset ✓✓✓
Pain with activities requiring gripping ✓✓✓
Localized or diffuse symptoms ✓✓✓

Objective:

Resisted wrist extension – pain ✓✓✓
Resisted extension of the middle finger in full elbow extension – pain ✓✓✓ (Fig 2.10)
Palpation – tenderness over ECRB tendon ✓✓✓

Special tests:

Upper limb neural provocation test 2b (ULNPT 2b) ✓ (Fig 2.11)

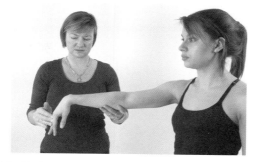

Fig 2.10   Resisted third finger extension.

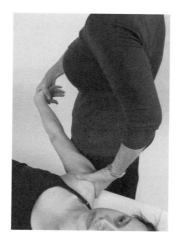

Fig 2.11   Upper limb neural provocation test 2b (radial nerve bias).

Associated injury:

Check no cervical spine involvement

Management:

Eccentric exercise programme (see Alfredson protocols for jumpers' knee and Achilles tendinopathy for frequency and duration of exercises, page 96)

Sport specific – check technique and racquet grip size, weight and string tension

Treat any neural/spinal involvement

Bracing – epicondylar clasp

Many more invasive treatments have been suggested when conservative management is unsuccessful (see Achilles tendinopathy) including injections (corticosteroid, autologous blood, sclerosant), extracorporeal shock wave therapy or surgery. The evidence regarding their efficacy is mixed

Medial elbow pain

Medial elbow pain can be separated into two different entities. The first involves overactivity of the wrist flexors and has been referred to as "golfer's elbow". The second has been more commonly termed "thrower's elbow". During this action, especially during the cocking and acceleration phases, the valgus load puts a stress on the MCL and compresses the radio-humeral joint.

"Golfer's" elbow

Subjective:

Pain with activity ✓✓✓ (golf or heavy top spin on the forehand in tennis)

Objective:

Resisted wrist flexion – pain ✓✓✓

Resisted pronation – pain ✓✓✓

Palpation – tenderness over medial epicondyle ✓✓✓

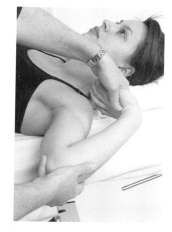

Fig 2.12 Upper limb neural provocation test 3 (ulnar nerve bias).

Special tests:

Upper limb neural provocation test 3 (ULNPT 3) (ulnar bias) ✓ (Fig 2.12)

Associated injury:

Check no cervical spine involvement

Management:

See lateral elbow pain

"Thrower's" elbow

Subjective:

Pain with activity ✓✓✓ (common in baseball pitchers and javelin throwers)

Objective:

Laxity ± pain with valgus stress test ✓✓ (Fig 2.13)

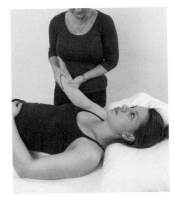

Fig 2.13 Valgus stress test for the medial collateral ligament of the elbow.

Associated injury:

Osteochondral damage to the radio-humeral joint

Management:

Sport specific – check technique
Taping
Strength and conditioning of forearm flexors and pronators

Wrist and hand

Triangular fibrocartilage complex (TFCC) injury

The TFCC is a small piece of cartilage that separates the ulna from the carpal bones and is integral to ulnar-carpal stability. Disruption to this complex may be acute or chronic. It occurs in high-velocity sports such as boxing and gymnastics, and hockey and racquet sports.

Subjective:

Pain on the ulnar side of the wrist with activity ✓✓✓
Clicking sound or sensation or clunking in the wrist ✓✓

Objective:

Ulnar swelling in the acute presentation ✓✓
Local tenderness ✓

Investigations:

MR Arthrography is the gold standard for diagnosis

Associated injury:

Differential diagnosis – extensor carpi ulnaris tear

Management:

Bracing
Arthroscopic surgical repair

Scaphoid–lunate dissociation

This is easy to miss and should be suspected in a case of chronic persistent wrist pain. It is caused by disruption of the scapholunate ligament and leads to instability/subluxation of the scaphoid, it is the most common carpal instability.

Subjective:

Acute traumatic episode ✓✓✓
Forced hyperextension of the wrist ± ulnar deviation ✓✓
Subsequent pain with activity ✓✓✓
Clicking/clunking in wrist ✓

Objective:

Tenderness over scapholunate border just distal to Lister's tubercle ✓✓✓
Grip strength – weakness ✓

Investigations:

Stress X-ray: AP view with a clenched fist reveals a gap between the lunate and scaphoid – the "Terry Thomas" sign in the presence of this condition ✓✓✓

2

Assessment and diagnosis of the injured athlete

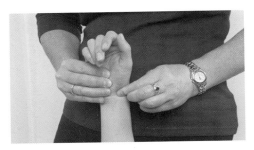

Fig 2.14 Scaphoid shift test for scapho-lunate ligamentous disruption.

Special tests:

Scaphoid shift test: palpate scaphoid tuberosity whilst moving the wrist from ulnar to radial deviation. This manoeuvre will be painful in this condition ✓✓ (Fig 2.14)

Associated injury:

Radial styloid fracture
Scaphoid fracture

Management:

Surgical repair. Delayed repair leads to degenerative changes

Skier's thumb

This used to be called gamekeeper's thumb and is a traumatic injury to the ulnar collateral ligament of the first metacarpal joint, now more often seen in skiers.

Subjective:

Fall where the thumb is forced into abduction and extension ✓✓✓

(The thumb can be forced into this direction during a fall whilst holding a ski pole or if the thumb gets caught in the strap of the pole)

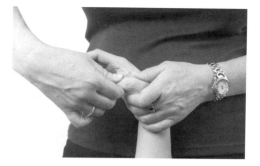

Fig 2.15 Valgus stress test for ulnar collateral ligament of the first metacarpal joint of the hand.

Immediate pain localized to the medial aspect of the thumb ✓✓✓

Objective:

Swelling

Valgus stress test (in flexion) – pain ± laxity ✓✓✓ (Fig 2.15)

Management:

Complete tear with excessive joint laxity requires surgical repair

Incomplete tear – immobilization with tape or splint for 4–6 weeks

Common Injuries in the Lower limb

Hip/groin and thigh

Groin pain

Groin pain is common in athletes especially in sports that involve twisting and kicking. Groin pain is also notoriously difficult to diagnose; symptoms are often recurrent and it is one of the major causes of lost playing time in sports like football and rugby. Many structures can be implicated and pathologies may co-exist, and there are no consistent patterns of presentation. Differential diagnosis includes hip joint pathology (labral pathology, chondral injury, osteoarthritis), inguinal hernia, adductor related pain (tendinopathy, enthesopathy, MT junction), nerve entrapment (ilioinguinal, obturator, genitofemoral), stress injury to the pubic bone, rectus abdominis strain, conjoint tendon tear, external oblique tear, iliopsoas syndrome, stress fracture neck of femur (NOF), referred lumbar pain (L1/2).

Subjective:

Pain:

Insidious or sudden onset

Localized or diffuse

Superficial or deep

Aggravated by activity ✓✓✓ NB: In many cases symptoms may have a latent response. Activity may not increase symptoms at the time, but an increased response is evident on objective testing

Objective:

Sensation – check

Hip range of motion (ROM) – can be reduced

Length and strength ± pain response (Table 2.2). Palpate where possible: resisted sit-up (rectus abdominis), adductor longus, iliopsoas, piriformis, trunk rotation (external oblique – opposite side)

Often poor lumbo-pelvic control – anterior tilt/increased hip flexion

Special tests:

FABER test (Fig 2.18)

Hip quadrant/labral grind test (Fig 2.19)

Femoral slump test

Table 2.2 Muscle tests for groin pain

Muscle	Length	Strength
Rectus abdominis	N/A	Sit-up
External oblique	N/A	Trunk rotation
Adductor longus	Often tight	Squeeze test (Fig 2.16) Resisted adduction in Thomas test position
Iliopsoas	Thomas test: often tight (Fig 2.17)	Hip flexion in Thomas test position
Piriformis	Often tight	

Valsalva manoeuvre – inguinal hernia

Hop test – stress fracture inferior pubic ramus

If few positive signs are elicited during the physical examination you may want to repeat the examination after training or competition.

Associated injury:

See differential diagnosis above – most common cause of groin pain in athletes is hip joint, pubic (males), psoas or adductor related pathology

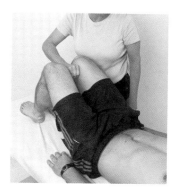

Fig 2.16 Squeeze tests for pubic overload. Note pain response. Use a pressure algometer to assess force.

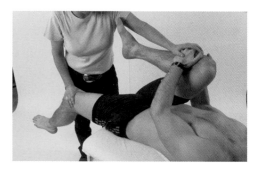

Fig 2.17 Thomas test.

Management:

Rehabilitation programme should be sign-driven, based on response to objective testing, rather than on symptom response

Stretch/mobilize any tight structures; correction of any muscle imbalance/fatigue/weakness issues (often gluteals/ hip abductor weakness) NB: Avoid stretching the adductor muscles. More effective to use soft tissue techniques to reduce tension in this muscle group

Graduated rehabilitation programme – with particular reference to progression from straight line to twisting activities

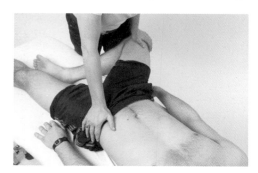

Fig 2.18 FABER test (**F**lexion / **AB**duction / **E**xternal **R**otation).

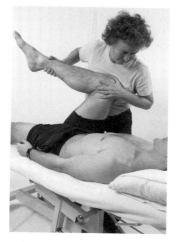

Fig 2.19 Hip quadrant test.

If no improvement after relative rest, correction of any dysfunction and graduated rehabilitation and return to play, investigations are warranted

Investigations:

MRI or LA injection, nerve conduction studies if indicated. Ultrasound is more sensitive for identifying tears to soft tissue structures in the abdominal wall

Falvey EC, Franklyn-Miller A and McCrory P (2009) The groin triangle: a patho-anatomical approach to the diagnosis of chronic groin pain in athletes. British Journal of Sports Medicine 43:213-220

Labral tear

Increasingly more recognized as a cause of pain in athletes in sports requiring turning, twisting and kicking. With improvements in MR imaging of the hip joint, increasing identification of labral tears is occurring. An anterior tear is the most common type and may present acutely or chronically. The symptoms can present in many different ways.

Subjective:

Pain maybe felt in either the groin/trochanteric/deep hip or low back ✓✓✓

Dull positional pain unrelated to activity ✓

Only provoked by activity ✓

Sharp catching pain ✓

Objective:

Quadrant test positive ✓✓ (see Fig 2.19)

FABER's test positive ✓✓ (see Fig 2.18)

NB: In the presence of hip pathology/dysfunction, hip flexion is often accompanied by a tendency for the hip to drift into abduction and external rotation. Also look for any pelvic tilt ✓✓✓

Investigations:

MRI/MRA to confirm diagnosis – but can be missed on scanning

Associated injury:

Iliopsoas dysfunction: positive Thomas test (see Fig 2.17)

Femoroacetabular impingement (FAI) whereby the femoral neck impinges against the acetabular labrum

These two conditions may co-exist or FAI may be a precursor to a labral tear

Differential diagnosis: femoral neck stress fracture if the athlete presents with an insidious onset of groin pain, with an increased index of suspicion with increased training loads or female endurance athletes with disordered eating and menstruation. Fulcrum test and bone scan to exclude this diagnosis

Management:

May resolve spontaneously. Unload the hip as necessary

In professional athletes the first line of treatment is arthroscopic debridement

Need to address biomechanical predisposing factors – anterior translation of femoral head – tight posterior hip capsule/overactive hip external rotators/poor gluteal function – tendency to perform hip external rotation rather than hip extension with gluteals/poor control of hip flexion by iliopsoas and overactive rectus femoris

Quads contusion (dead leg)

Common in contact sports such as rugby. Need to differentiate between a direct blow and a strain. Management for a strain is similar. In young athletes proximal anterior thigh pain may be an avulsion at the apophysis of rectus femoris.

Subjective:

Direct blow to the thigh ✓✓✓

Objective:

Localized anterior thigh pain ✓✓✓

Swelling ✓✓✓

Resisted quads: pain ✓✓✓

Prone passive quads stretch – painful and limited ✓✓✓ (Fig 2.20). NB: Less than 90° knee flexion indicates that the player is likely to be out for several weeks

Special tests:

Single leg hop – pain and reduced performance

Squat – pain

Management:

Remove from the field of play

PRICE and NWB on crutches if necessary

No aggressive treatment locally to haematoma – risk of re-bleed up to 10 days

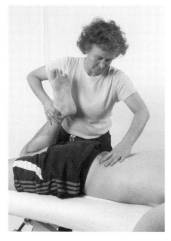

Fig 2.20 Passive stretch / length test for quadriceps (include hip extension if necessary).

Isometric quads (pain free) initially
Passive quads stretch (aim to have rectus femoris test R=L)
Beware of myositis ossificans in unresolving signs and symptoms

Hamstring strain

Common in sports involving sprinting, especially track sprinters, football, rugby and Australian rules. Usually occurs proximally and laterally – biceps femoris ✓✓
The aetiology is multifactoral, the only factors that are predictors for this injury are age and previous hamstring injury. The risk of recurrence is up to 30%.

Subjective:

Sudden onset posterior thigh pain during explosive sprint ✓✓✓
Unable to continue ✓✓

Objective:

Bruising ✓✓

Locally sore on palpation ✓✓✓

Palpable gap with complete rupture ✓✓✓

Gait: reduced stride length ✓✓

Passive knee extension (PKE) test: limited and painful ✓✓✓ (Fig 2.21)

Resisted knee flexion pain ± weakness ✓✓✓

Resisted tibial lateral rotation (at 90° flexion) pain ± weakness ✓

Investigations:

Ultrasound imaging diagnostic within the first 24 hours after injury

MRI-diagnostic after 24 hours

Special tests:

Unable to accelerate ✓✓✓

Referred pain can mimic this injury and a neural component is often present; check the lumbar spine and clear the slump test (sciatic nerve) ✓✓ (Fig 2.22)

Lumbo-pelvic dysfunction often present

   – Hamstrings overactive relative to gluteals

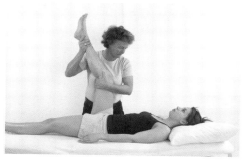

Fig 2.21 Passive knee extension test.

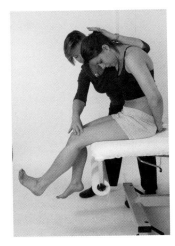

Fig 2.22 Slump test.

- Erector spinae overactive relative to gluteals (Fig 2.23)
- Timing issues

Management: (see also Case Study in Section 3 p 189)
Initially PRICE and NWB with crutches if necessary
Active and passive exercises to increase ROM

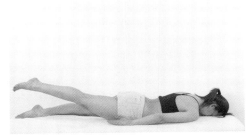

Fig 2.23 Prone hip extension demonstrating relative erector spinae and gluteal activity.

Isometric (pain free exercises) as soon as this can be tolerated, progressing to isotonic (concentric)

Proximal stability work

Nordic hamstring eccentric training programme (see Fig 3.21a,b)

Week 1	×1	2 sets × 5 reps
Week 2	×2	2 sets × 6 reps
Week 3	×3	3 sets × 6–8 reps
Week 4	×3	3 sets × 8–12 reps
Week 5	×3	3 sets × 8–12 reps

End stage agility, sports specific and Return to Play (RTP) evaluations must be completed (see Section 4).

Knee

Acute knee injuries

After any traumatic knee injury it is important to establish the nature and behaviour of the swelling as this is indicative of certain diagnoses. If the whole knee swells immediately (i.e. within a couple of hours) this is indicative of a haemarthrosis. The cause must be one of the following intra-articular structures – anterior/posterior cruciate ligaments (ACL/PCL), meniscus or osteochondral. Swelling by the following morning is more indicative of a synovitis which presents with a degenerative meniscus or articular cartilage injury.

The sensitivity of some of the objective tests will be affected by the degree of swelling present at the time of examination.

Anterior cruciate ligament (ACL) injury

Common injury in football, rugby and skiing. In the presence of a haemarthrosis there is a 75% chance of ACL involvement, so suspect this until proven otherwise.

Subjective:

Classic history of a twisting injury, sudden change of direction with knee flexion and valgus, non-contact, ended up on the floor ✓✓✓

Often describe a popping sound ✓✓
Immediate swelling (lasts 4–6 weeks) ✓✓✓
Unable to play on ✓✓✓
Subsequent feeling of instability or episodes of giving way in the absence of pain ✓✓✓

Objective:
Active and passive extension – limited ✓✓✓
Active and passive flexion – limited ✓✓
Lachmann's test – increased laxity ✓✓✓ (Fig 2.24)
Pivot shift or jerk test – positive ✓✓ (This test is difficult to learn and if an athlete has a positive test it is unlikely they will allow you to repeat this. The best way to learn this test is in an operating theatre) (Fig 2.25)

Associated Injury:
Medial collateral ligament (MCL), meniscus (medial more common), bone bruising in 75–90% of cases

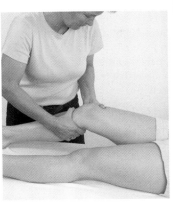 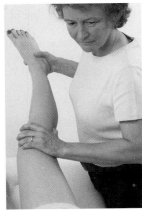

Fig 2.24 Lachmann's test for the integrity of the ACL.

Fig 2.25 Pivot shift test.

Management:

Consider surgical reconstruction in the professional athlete and high-demand sports. Otherwise, a conservative rehabilitation programme should be instigated and only failure of this (episodes of knee giving way) would indicate the need for surgery

Medial collateral ligament (MCL) injury

More commonly injured than the lateral collateral ligament (LCL). Occurs frequently in skiing, football and rugby

Subjective:

Valgus force (a blow to the outside) to the knee or twisting ✓✓✓
Medial pain ✓✓
Medial swelling ✓

Objective:

Limited ROM ✓✓✓
Valgus testing at 20° knee flexion – pain ± laxity ✓✓✓ (Fig 2.26)
Palpation – pain ✓✓

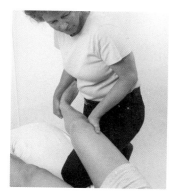

Fig 2.26 Valgus testing of the knee for medial collateral ligament integrity.

Associated injury:

Medial meniscus with a twisting mechanism

Management: (see also Case Study in Section 3 p 202)

PRICE

Grade 2/3:

- MRI to assess associated injury
- Brace with a block to the last 20° extension for 2–4 weeks

Progressive rehabilitation programme

Meniscal injury

The medial meniscus is injured more frequently than the lateral one in acute knee injuries. It commonly occurs in twisting sports such as football, rugby and basketball.

Subjective:

Twisting injury on a fixed foot ✓✓✓

Immediate swelling with a peripheral tear, delayed in a central or degenerative tear ✓✓✓

Subsequent locking ✓✓ Player may or may not be able to unlock the knee

Feeling of instability ✓✓

Localized pain with activity ✓✓✓

Objective:

Passive extension – block ✓✓✓

Passive flexion – painful ✓✓

Joint line palpation – pain ✓✓

Special tests:

McMurray's has traditionally been advocated as the test for meniscal injuries, but it is neither sensitive nor specific.

Pain on palpation of the medial joint line has been shown to be a more reliable indicator of medial meniscal injury. ✓

Squatting ✓

Associated injury:

ACL, MCL, chondral injury

Management:

In symptomatic athletes – arthroscopy and repair or partial meniscectomy

Post-operative rehabilitation programme

Posterior cruciate ligament (PCL) injury

Less frequently injured than the ACL and tends to cause fewer problems when it is injured. These injuries are commonly missed because of a lack of pain and functional restriction. It is often diagnosed incorrectly as an ACL lesion because an anterior drawer test can appear positive. They can present chronically with patients reporting vague, diffuse symptoms of pain, often in the anterior knee region

Subjective:

Blow to the anterior tibia on a semi-flexed knee ✓✓✓ – "dashboard injury"

Fall onto the front of a flexed knee

Pain and swelling – minimal compared to ACL ✓✓

Objective:

Posterior tibial sag ✓✓✓

Fewer symptoms of instability than in ACL injuries – vague feeling of unsteadiness

Associated injury:

Structures in the posterolateral corner – check dial test (Fig 2.27)

Management:

Some orthopaedic surgeons advocate the use of an extension brace in the early stages of rehabilitation to prevent the posterior sagging of the tibia relative to the femur

2

Assessment and diagnosis of the injured athlete

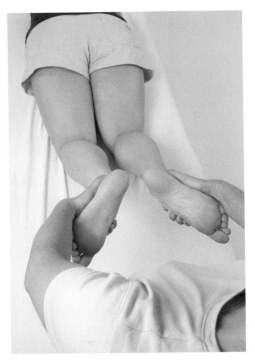

Fig 2.27 Dial test for integrity of the posterolateral corner of the knee.

Conservative rehabilitation programme with an emphasis on the quadriceps

Surgery – only recommended for Grade 3 tears – and even then this is somewhat controversial

Chronic or overuse knee injuries

Patellofemoral or anterior knee pain

This condition is common in adolescents, females and endurance runners. No clear agreement exists as to the cause of pain. Evidence suggests it is multifactoral in nature with lower limb biomechanical dysfunction leading to patellar maltracking.

Subjective:

Pain – anterior but not well localized ✓✓✓

Pain aggravated by running and stairs (predominantly down) and prolonged sitting with the knee bent ✓✓✓

Insidious onset ✓✓

With an acute history it often occurs following prolonged downhill walking or running ✓✓

Sensation of instability but not true giving way ✓✓

Locking ✓

Objective:

Biomechanical: Excessive pronation ✓

Poor flexibility: iliotibial band (ITB) (Fig 2.28), hamstrings (see Fig 2.21), gastrocnemius and rectus femoris (see Fig 2.20) ✓✓

2

Assessment and diagnosis of the injured athlete

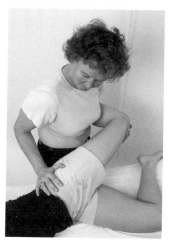

Fig 2.28 Ober's test for ITB tightness.

Gluteus medius – weak ✓✓
Functional testing – single leg stance/small knee bend
VMO delayed onset prior to vastus lateralis ✓✓

Functional testing

When examining patients with chronic, overuse or biomechanical problems, it is essential to establish a direct relationship between the presence of poor biomechanical features and the individual patient's symptoms. This can be easily achieved by following this simple process:

1. Identify a functional movement or specific test that provokes the patient's symptoms (in this case anterior knee pain)
2. Identify the poor biomechanical features present
3. Alter **one** of these features – e.g. facilitate VMO function/activate gluteus medius to control hip internal rotation/support the foot to prevent over-pronation – while the patient repeats the functional movement
4. Note the effect on the patient's symptoms

If no change is noted in the patient's symptoms, it is unlikely that correcting this biomechanical feature is going to have a marked effect on the patient's symptoms.
Repeat this process, identifying those biomechanical corrections that improve symptoms.
Focus treatment on manual techniques and exercises that correct these biomechanical faults.

Special tests:
Ober's test – positive ✓✓ (see Fig 2.28)
FABER test (see Fig 2.18)
Assessment of patella position – tilted and/or rotated
Slump test (femoral nerve)
Step down test ✓✓✓
Thomas test (see Fig 2.17) – note effect of altering P/F position and T/F rotation

Associated injury:
Fat pad impingement
Tibiofemoral dysfunction

Management:

Correct biomechanics – orthotics for excessive pronation, short-term bracing or taping to correct maltracking

Re-education of VMO and gluteus medius in functional closed kinetic chain programme. Good proximal control

Stretch any tight structures – ITB, hamstrings, gastrocnemius, rectus femoris

Patella tendinopathy

Otherwise known as "jumper's knee", it is common in basketball and athletic field events. Due to the nature of the symptoms, players can often play through the early stages of this and (as with other tendinopathies) they can become chronic and recalcitrant (see Achilles tendinopathy). The cause of the symptoms remains unclear; however it is known not to be due to an inflammatory process, and may be the result of a failed healing response.

Subjective:

Anterior knee pain – localized to the tendon ✓✓✓

Initially comes on after aggravating activity, then during but does not limit activity. Eventually restricts activity ✓✓✓

Objective:

Tender on palpation of the inferior pole of the patella (common location) ✓✓✓

Swelling ✓

Decreased muscle length: gastrocnemius/ hamstring ✓

Biomechanical evaluation

Investigations:

Diagnostic US reveals hypoechoic areas and neovascularization (Fig 2.29)

Special tests:

Eccentric loading: single leg squats (with additional weight if necessary) ✓✓

2

Assessment and diagnosis of the injured athlete

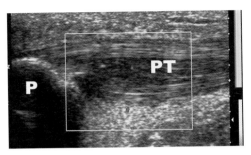

Fig 2.29 Ultrasound showing hypoechoic region in the patella tendon (PT).

Management:

Reduction of abusive load – activity modification

Conditioning of quadriceps and gastrocnemius

Eccentric rehabilitation programme (after Alfredson et al 1998): single leg on a decline squat (Fig 2.30), 3 sets of

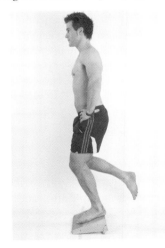

Fig 2.30 Eccentric training on a decline board for patella tendinopathy.

15 repetitions, twice a day for 12 weeks (into pain). Increase load as symptoms resolve. Large volume (i.e. number of repetitions) is considered important in effectively managing this condition

Failed rehabilitation programme – alternative approaches – sclerosant injection, shockwave therapy, GTN patches, microcurrent therapy, surgical decompression

Iliotibial band (ITB) syndrome

Lateral knee pain around the lateral epicondyle of the femur is a common condition in long-distance runners and is thought to be caused by the ITB rubbing against this prominence with repeated knee flexion and extension.

Subjective:

Pain with running especially running on steeper cambers and downhill ✓✓✓

Able to run pain free with straight leg ✓✓

Objective:

Local tenderness over lateral condyle ✓✓✓

Gait: over pronation ✓✓

Hip abduction weak ✓✓

Special tests:

Ober's test positive ✓✓✓ (see Fig 2.28)

Modified Ober's test positive ✓✓✓

Associated injury:

A tight ITB is often associated with patellofemoral pain (which can also present as lateral knee pain)

Differential diagnosis from a lateral meniscal lesion and patellofemoral pain is usually by location of the pain

Management:

Modification/reduction of training load

Correct any abnormal biomechanics

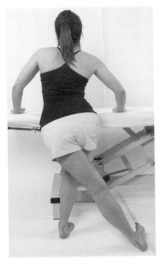 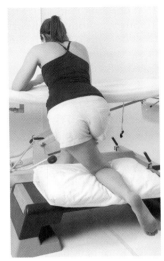

Fig 2.31 ITB stretch in standing.   **Fig 2.32** ITB stretch in kneeling.

Re-education of proximal control around hip with special attention to hip abduction and external rotation

Stretch ITB (Figs 2.31 and 2.32)

ITB: myofascial and trigger point work, dry needling

Graduated return to running (refer to Section 3 for more details)

Consider injection therapy in recalcitrant cases

Lower leg and ankle

Leg pain in sport

Exercise-induced leg pain is a common cause of disability in all running athletes and traditionally this has been referred to as "shin splints". However, this is a complete misnomer as it does not help differentiate where the pain is coming from and the clinician should consider whether the origin is:

Bony – tibial stress fracture

Tenoperiosteal – medial tibial stress syndrome (MTSS)

Muscular – chronic exertional compartment syndrome (CECS).

In all three conditions the subject will complain of pain over the medial and anterior tibial border. A detailed history, site of pain and the behaviour of the symptoms will help in the differential diagnosis. Clinically they do not always present as discrete entities and there may be overlap in presentation. Exclude any neural involvement (common peroneal-tibial nerve) in all cases.

Tibial stress fracture

Bone stress injuries result in significant loss/modification of training in many different types of athlete. They are common in runners and endurance athletes and may be associated with disordered eating and irregular menstruation in female athletes. There is often a delay in diagnosis until the pain becomes severe enough to warrant investigation.

Subjective:

Mostly unilateral ✓✓✓

Pain over medial tibial border (lower 1/3 and upper 2/3) ✓✓✓

Increasing or "crescendo" pain with activity ✓✓✓

Pain at rest and at night in more advanced cases ✓✓

Training mileage > 50 miles/week ✓✓

Objective:

Local swelling, tenderness and pinpoint pain ✓✓✓

Biomechanics: over-pronation or a supinated foot ✓✓

Investigations:

Isotope bone scan/MRI for a positive diagnosis

Special tests:

Tuning fork over the suspected area will reproduce pain ✓✓

Management:

Load reduction protocol – no provocative activity for up to 6 weeks. Graduated return to weight-bearing activity, this can be started in a pool where initial load-bearing can be controlled. Improve flexibility in the posterior muscle groups in the lower limb

New therapies are now advocated for the management of bone stress injuries and these include: biphosphonates (controversial especially in young women), hyperbaric oxygen therapy, electromagnetic field stimulation, ultrasound, growth factors, bone morphogenic protein (BMPs) and parathyroid hormone

Medial tibial stress syndrome (MTSS)

Subjective:

Mostly unilateral but can be bilateral ✓✓

Pain over medial tibial border (lower 1/3) ✓✓✓

Sudden increase in training intensity or change of surface ✓✓

Initially pain starts with onset of exercise and wears off after warming up ✓✓✓

Pain after activity and at rest ✓✓✓

Objective:

Palpation – tender medial border lower 1/3 tibia ✓✓✓

Biomechanical evaluation: excessive pronation or supinated foot ✓✓

Poor proximal functional control with reduced core stability and lumbo-pelvic control is frequently seen ✓✓

Possible positive neural provocation at the lumbosacral level

Investigations:

Isotope bone scan/MRI for grading of the tibial stress injury

Management: (see also Case Study in Section 3 p 207)

Address any biomechanical abnormalities – restrict excessive pronation, improve shock absorption for a supinated foot. Use tape and felt to determine any effect on symptoms

For further information see Vicenzino B (2004) Foot orthotics in the treatment of lower limb conditions: a musculoskeletal physiotherapy perspective. Manual Therapy 9(4):185-196

Soft tissue and manual therapy techniques

Alter training surface

Where conservative management is unsuccessful, consider injection and possible periosteal stripping

Chronic exertional compartment syndrome (CECS)

There are four compartments in the lower leg. The anterior compartment is the most commonly affected but other sections can be involved. CECS of the deep posterior compartment can mimic MTSS.

Subjective:

Usually bilateral ✓✓✓

Pain on exercise which completely subsides with rest (within minutes) ✓✓✓

Sudden increase in training load ✓

Objective:

At rest – usually normal ✓✓✓

Exercise – provocative exercise will produce symptoms ✓✓✓

Sometimes there may be a presence of muscle hernia ✓

Special tests:

Dynamic intra-compartmental pressure (DICP) measurements (ICPs) – a catheter is inserted into the relevant compartment and the subject runs on a treadmill.

Normal resting pressures 0–15 mmHg; in CECS this may elevate resting pressure to 20–25 mmHg and, average exercise pressure to > 35 mmHg ✓✓✓

Management:

Once the diagnosis is confirmed with a good history and objective DICP evidence, surgery offers the best solution. Consider superficial fasciotomy first and, failing that, a fasciectomy may be required

Post-operative management is important, early mobilization as tolerated and soft tissue work and neural mobilizations. Progress to sport specific rehab at 3–4 weeks

Gastrocnemius tear (tennis calf)

Occurs at the musculotendinous junction of the medial calf in middle-aged recreational tennis and squash players

Subjective:

Sudden lunge, drive, reaching for the ball ✓✓✓
Common description "felt like I had been shot" ✓✓✓
Unable to play on ✓✓✓
Localized pain ✓✓

Objective:

Localized swelling ✓✓
Gait: reduced stride length ✓✓✓
Resisted plantarflexion – painful ✓✓✓
Passive dorsiflexion (knee in full extension) – painful ✓✓

Special test:

Single leg heel raise – pain ✓✓✓

Associated Injury:

Neural involvement may be present – check slump test (see Fig 2.22)

Management:

PRICE

Grade 3 tear: immobilize in plantarflexion in a heel walker for 2 weeks and then follow a progressive rehabilitation programme

Achilles tendinopathy (AT)

The "curse" of the running athlete (especially track athletes). Occurs mostly in the mid-portion of the tendon and this is most amenable to conservative treatment. Insertional AT into the calcaneum is more difficult to manage and is not covered below. The cause of the pain is still unclear; but research has established that it is not an inflammatory condition.

Subjective:

Gradual onset ✓✓✓

Initially pain after exercise, progresses to pain during ✓✓✓

Pain and stiffness immediately on waking ✓✓✓

Poor and/or a sudden change in training techniques: increased load, reduced recovery time ✓✓

Objective:

Tender on palpation ✓✓✓

Thickened tendon ✓✓

Poor biomechanics; increased pronation ✓✓

Tight gastrocnemius/soleus ✓✓

Reduced ankle dorsiflexion ✓✓

Investigations:

Diagnostic ultrasound will reveal a hypoechoic tendon (see Fig 2.29) and the presence of neovascularization

Special tests:

Neural involvement: tibial nerve

Management:

Modify training load

Twelve-week eccentric training programme (Alfredson et al 1998) 3 sets 15 reps, twice a day for 12 weeks (Fig 2.33a–d). To start, raise up onto tiptoes using the unaffected leg, then heel drop over the edge of the step on the affected leg only. Alternate between knee bent and straight. When exercises become pain free, add load using a rucksack so they provoke pain again. Progress weight up to 60 kg

Alfredson H, Pietila T, Jonsson P et al (1998) Heavy-load eccentric calf muscle training for the treatment of chronic Achilles tendinosis. American Journal of Sports Medicine 26:360-366

Correct any abnormal biomechanics and consider use of a heel raise to offload the tendon

Strength and conditioning of calf complex, stretch and mobilize any tight structures

Graduated controlled return to activity

Failed conservative treatment: surgical strip, high-volume injection, sclerosant injection

Partial Achilles tendon rupture

Often mistaken for Achilles tendinopathy due to similarities in the clinical presentation. Individuals with partial ruptures have more subtle symptoms of weakness and changes in resting tone than cases of total tendon rupture. A misdiagnosis as tendinopathy and treatment with an eccentric exercise programme can result in an extension of the tear and lengthening of the tendon. Accurate diagnosis is essential, but not easy.

Subjective:

Sudden onset or significant increase in pain in the Achilles tendon during running or walking ✓✓✓

Sudden onset or increase in pain may occur in the presence of chronic low-level pain ✓✓

Subtle feeling of weakness in calf/Achilles region ✓✓

Objective:

Thickening and tenderness in the midportion of the Achilles tendon ✓✓✓

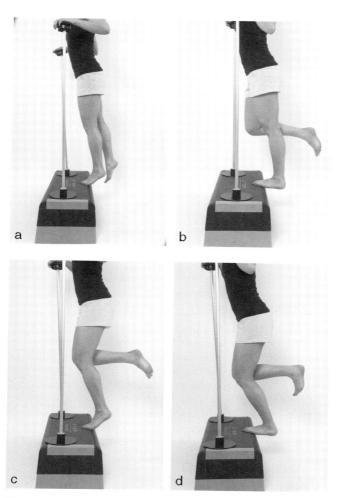

Fig 2.33 Eccentric training programme for Achilles tendinopathy (Alfredson et al 1998): (a) start position, knee straight; (b) finish position, knee straight; (c) start position, knee bent; (d) finish position, knee bent.

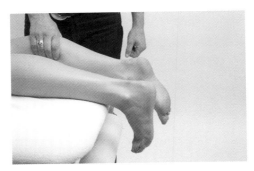

Fig 2.34 – Simmond's test (also called Thomson's test) for rupture of the Achilles tendon.

Reduced resting tone of the foot in prone, compared to the uninjured foot. This sign is more subtle than utilizing Thomson's test (see Fig 2.34) ✓✓

Resisted plantarflexion – weak and painful ✓✓✓

Painful weakness during tendon loading (attempted eccentric programme) ✓✓✓

NB: These physical findings are very similar to those present in athletes with Achilles tendinopathy; however athletes with Achilles tendinopathy DO NOT demonstrate changes in resting tone and weakness. Any patient not responding to an eccentric programme or experiencing extreme levels of pain while performing these exercises should be referred to a clinician with expertise in the management of Achilles tendon pain who can examine the tendon with colour Doppler ultrasound

Investigations:

Ultrasound imaging usually shows disruption of the tendon along the superficial/dorsal aspect (closest to the skin) of the midportion of the tendon. This is seen as irregular tendon structure on ultrasound ✓✓

Colour Doppler imaging – high blood flow in the superficial aspect of the tendon

NB: This contrasts with the ultrasound findings in tendinopathy where the majority of the structural and blood flow changes are seen in the deep/ventral aspect of the tendon

Alfredson HA, Masci L and Öhberg I (2011) Partial midportion Achilles tendon rupture: new sonographic findings helpful for diagnosis. British Journal of Sports Medicine 45:429-432

Management:

Elite athletes with recurrent or ongoing symptoms – consider surgical repair

Conservative management:
- use of heel lift for 3 months
- avoidance of loaded dorsiflexion activities/impact for 3 months

Achilles tendon rupture

More common in middle-aged (30−50 years) male squash and badminton players.

Subjective:

Often injured during a lunge for the ball/shuttle ✓✓✓

Athlete describes a sound like a shot gun going off ✓✓

Feels as though they have been kicked in the back of the leg ✓✓✓

Often not very painful following complete rupture ✓✓✓

Unable to "push off" ✓✓✓

Objective:

Shortened stride length ✓✓✓

NB: look at resting tone in prone. Foot lies in less plantar-flexion than uninjured foot

Resisted plantarflexion – weak ✓✓✓

Single leg heel raise – unable to do ✓✓✓

Palpation: palpable gap 3–6 cm above the insertion into the calcaneum ✓✓ (depends on the time of examination following injury)

Special tests:

Simmond's, squeeze or Thomson's test ✓✓✓ (Fig 2.34)

Note: some plantarflexion will be possible via tibialis posterior, flexor hallucis and digitorum longus

Management:

Lack of consensus and depends on the demands of the athlete

Surgical repair in younger athletes, but complications associated with surgery other than re-rupture

Conservative management: functional bracing leads to shorter rehabilitation than immobilization in a cast. Conservative management associated with higher rates of re-rupture

Tibialis posterior tendinopathy/dysfunction

The tendon can be affected at various sites along its complex path. Occurs more commonly behind the medial malleolus or at the insertion towards the navicular. In management, it is important to control dynamic stability of the foot since tibialis posterior dysfunction will have an adverse effect on foot biomechanics.

Subjective:

Insidious onset medial ankle pain ✓✓

Aggravated by activity ✓✓✓

Objective:

Tenderness and swelling along the tendon ✓✓

Resisted inversion – painful ± weakness ✓✓✓

Passive eversion – painful ✓✓

Altered biomechanics: increased pronation ✓✓

Special tests:

Single leg heel raise – pain ✓✓

Management:

Correct biomechanics:
– Orthotics
– Proximal hip control
– Intrinsic muscle strength
– Strengthen tibialis posterior – eccentric control of
  pronation through arch

Ankle sprain

This is one of the most common acute sporting injuries with
a high recurrence rate. It is frequently seen in football, rugby
and basketball. The anterior talofibular ligament (ATFL) is
the most commonly injured of the lateral ligament complex,
followed by the calcaneofibular and the posterior talofibular
ligament, respectively.

Subjective:

Mechanism: "went over on my ankle" normally non-contact
forced inversion and plantarflexion, resulting in lateral pain
and swelling ✓✓✓
Bruising after 24–48 hours ✓✓

Objective:

Active and passive inversion – pain ✓✓✓ (Fig 2.35)
Palpation – tender over insertion or origin of ATFL ✓✓
Weight-bearing – pain ✓

Investigations:

X-Ray if lateral malleolar or base of 5th metatarsal fracture
suspected

Special tests:

Anterior draw test ✓✓✓ for complete rupture of ATFL
Talar tilt test for calcaneofibular ligament injury
Neural involvement: common peroneal nerve

2

Assessment and diagnosis of the injured athlete

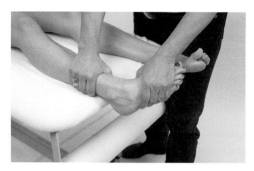

Fig 2.35 Test for ATFL ligament laxity or sprain (plantarflexion and inversion).

Associated injury:

Be suspicious if intra-articular swelling develops and consider associated talar dome injury. Consider sinus tarsi syndrome, syndesmosis injury or other diagnoses in an unresolving ankle sprain

Management: (see also Case Study in Section 3 p 179)
PRICE
Normalize gait if affected – PWB/NWB with crutches
Refer to proprioception section in Section 3 – emphasis on proprioception
Functional braces are often used for protection during the rehabilitation period, but there is no evidence to suggest these prevent recurrence or chronic ankle instability (CAI)

Ankle impingement

Ankle impingement may occur posteriorly, and this is common in sports that require repetitive and forced plantarflexion such as football, gymnastics, and

dancing. Impingement (the so called "footballers ankle")
may also occur anteriorly or simultaneously.

	Anterior	**Posterior**
Subjective:	Anterior pain ✓✓✓	Posterior pain ✓✓✓
	Exacerbated by activity ✓✓✓	
Objective:		
Palpation - tender	Anterior joint line ✓✓✓	Deep posteriorly ✓✓
	Restricted DF ✓✓	
Special tests:		Impingement test +ve ✓✓✓ (Fig 2.36)

Investigations:

X-ray frequently shows osteophytes on the tibia and talus in
anterior impingement

Associated injury:

Differential diagnosis with posterior impingement include:
enlarged posterior talar tubercle, os trigonum and Haglund's
deformity

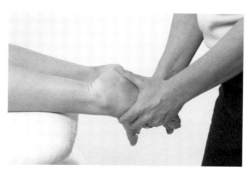

Fig 2.36   Ankle posterior impingement test.

2

Assessment and diagnosis of the injured athlete

Management:

Manual mobilization to the talocrural and subtalar joints, soft tissue work, taping and/or orthotics, technique modification – especially for ballet dancers
Where conservative methods fail, a corticosteroid injection may be warranted or arthroscopic removal of loose bodies or surgical management of the differential diagnoses

Lisfranc injury

This refers to the tarsometatarsal joint of the foot and can present as anything from a mild sprain to fracture/dislocation between the first and second metatarsal. It is often misdiagnosed. If missed, there is a high risk of chronic secondary disability.

Subjective:

Mid foot pain ✓✓✓

Trauma or insidious onset. Mechanism of injury – axial loading in extreme plantar flexion ✓✓✓

Often seen in jumping/landing on toes (rugby players) or during push-off while sprinting

Weight-bearing – pain, unable to run ✓✓✓

Objective:

Unable to weight bear on toes ✓✓✓

Localized swelling ✓✓

Positive squeeze test ✓✓

Focal tenderness ✓✓✓

Fix calcaneum, passive eversion and abduction is painful ✓✓

Hypermobility 1st ray – more chronic condition

Investigations:

Plain weight-bearing X-rays to exclude fracture/dislocation if suspected. NB. Must be weight-bearing to see ligamentous disruption (Fig 2.37)

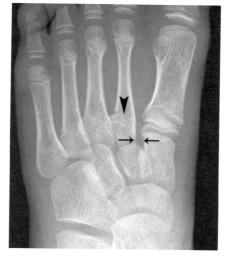

Fig 2.37 X-ray showing Lisfranc injury.

Special tests:

Check dorsalis pedis artery is not compromised.

Management:

Depends on the severity of injury: non-weight-bearing cast in cases with no disruption. Surgical intervention is necessary for fracture/dislocation

Navicular stress fracture

Common in track athletes and dancers. The central third of the navicular is relatively avascular, so is prone to delayed or non-union

Subjective:

Pain is associated with training – onset gradually occurs earlier into activity ✓✓✓

Objective:

Palpation elicits local tenderness over the proximal dorsal part of the navicular – "N" spot ✓✓

Cavus foot ✓✓

Short first metatarsal or long second metatarsal ✓✓

Hop test – painful ✓

Toe walking – painful ✓

Investigations:

Isotope bone scan or CT to confirm diagnosis

Management:

Non weight-bearing cast for 6 weeks is successful in the majority of cases

Some clinicians advocate the use of a walking boot – to reduce a loss of function

Surgical intervention should be considered if conservative management fails and there is non-union of the fracture

See tibial stress fracture (page 91) for new therapies for stress fractures

Turf toe

This is a hyperextension injury of the 1st MTP joint disrupting the plantar capsule and ligament. This has been increasingly seen in football players since the inception of artificial pitches.

Subjective:

Forced hyperextension of the 1st MTP ✓✓✓. Player may not be able to recall specific incident

Pain on weight-bearing and push-off ✓✓✓

Objective:

Tenderness on palpation ✓✓✓

Passive extension 1st MTP – painful ✓✓✓

Management:

PRICE offload the foot – NWB or PWB as tolerated

Ensure full extension of the 1st MTP is regained as healing time allows or function and performance will be compromised. Full extension is necessary to gain maximum propulsion during gait

Sesamoiditis

Caused by inflammation of the sesamoid bones under the first MTP joint.

Subjective:

Pain under the ball of the foot on weight-bearing ✓✓✓

Objective:

Tender on palpation of the sesamoids ✓✓

Resisted plantarflexion of the 1st toe –painful ✓✓✓

Investigations:

MRI to exclude stress fracture or bipartite sesamoid

Management:

Offload the area – look at footwear. Possible use of orthotics in the presence of abnormal biomechanics. Usually self-resolving

Blisters

Blisters are the most common overuse sporting injury and are caused by friction of the skin against an interface that could be clothing, shoes or equipment.

Management:

The best management is prevention – wear well-fitting socks that wick moisture to keep feet as dry as possible, wear-in new shoes gradually, alternate use with an older pair and apply zinc oxide tape to areas that are rubbing. If the skin is already red and activity has to be continued, apply a

2

Assessment and diagnosis of the injured athlete

hydrocolloid dressing. In the case of hands, wear hand protection/gloves, e.g. golf, sailing and wheelchair athletics. If a blister has already formed, remove the cause of friction if possible and treat with tape or hydrocolloid dressing. Do not burst a fluid-filled blister unless this is absolutely necessary as it will be vulnerable to infection. If this must be done to alleviate pain or facilitate mobility, use an aseptic technique, leave the skin intact and treat with antibiotic ointment. If the blister has burst spontaneously, apply an antiseptic/antibiotic application and dressings

Examination of the spinal region

Introduction

When dealing with athletes experiencing spinal pain and other symptoms, the most essential aspect of your examination is to identify those individuals with serious underlying pathology, such as tumours, infections or fractures, as a source of their pain. It is not uncommon for clinicians to assume that "fit and healthy" athletes are just that, and discount the possibility of some underlying systemic or sinister pathology.

It is commonly accepted that, in searching for the existence of serious spinal pathology, the identification of "red flags" is crucial. The majority of "red flags" are symptoms and therefore, a detailed and probing subjective examination is the most important aspect of the examination. The existing evidence would suggest that physical signs are less reliable in determining the presence of sinister pathology, hence the importance of the subjective examination.

As well as excluding sinister spinal pathology in your subjective questioning, you should also investigate for non-spinal causes of neck and back pain including spondyloarthropathies and other inflammatory conditions. These conditions are often associated with the presence of other physical signs and symptoms such as rashes or enthesopathies and require further investigations and interventions from the medical team. Other non-spinal causes of pain include visceral problems and pathology. You should question the athlete to ensure they do not have any other general health problems or other symptoms that may be associated with these conditions.

A list of subjective questions for "red flags" and non-spinal causes of neck and back pain can be found in the box below.

Questions relating to suspected serious pathology

- Is the athlete aged under 20 or over 55?
- Is there any evidence of violent trauma that may suggest structural damage?
- Is there a lack of specific aggravating and easing factors? Are they ever free of pain? Does their pain alter with movement?
- Do they have a persistent structural deformity or widespread limitation of movement in both the spine and limbs? Are they very stiff in the mornings?
- Do they ever have pain at night or at rest?
- Do they have any significant past history – Cancer/HIV/inflammatory problems of other structures?
- Do they have any significant family history?
- Have they any evidence of steroid use/abuse/other drug abuse?
- Is the athlete unwell is any other way? Presence of flu-like symptoms/lethargy/gut disturbances/rashes?
- Has there been any recent change in their body weight? Is there a reasonable explanation for this?
- Do they have any areas of pins and needles/numbness?
- Do they have problems with their bowel or bladder function?
- Have they noted any problems with their balance or feelings of weakness in their limbs?

The potential for neurological compromise must also be determined in the examination, including testing of sensation (Fig 2.38), muscle power and reflexes. Specific testing techniques can be found in most texts dealing with examination of the musculoskeletal system and will not be repeated here; however Fig 2.39a-l illustrates quick screening tests for the muscle power in both the upper and lower limbs.

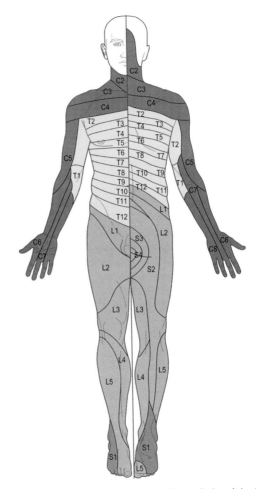

Fig 2.38 Dermatomes of the upper and lower limbs. Adapted from Kenyon – *Pocketbook of Physiotherapy*, with permission.

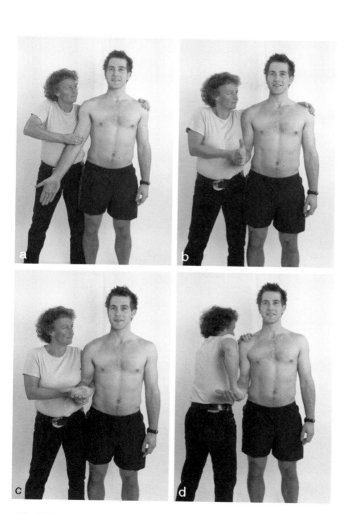

Fig 2.39a-l Myotomal testing for upper limb and lower limb: (a) resisted shoulder abduction (C5), (b) resisted shoulder external rotation (C5/6), (c) resisted elbow extension (C7), (d) resisted elbow flexion (C6),

(Continued)

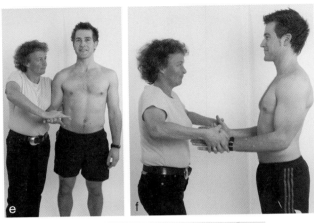

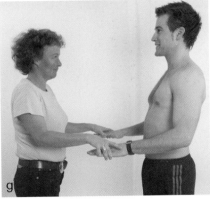

Fig 2.39—cont'd (e) resisted wrist extension (C7), (f) resisted thumb extension (C8), (g) resisted finger abduction (T1),

(Continued)

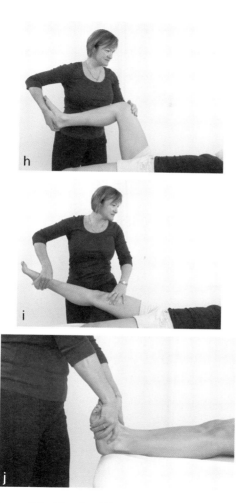

Fig 2.39—cont'd (h) resisted hip flexion (L2), (i) resisted knee extension (L3), (j) resisted ankle dorsiflexion (L4),

(Continued)

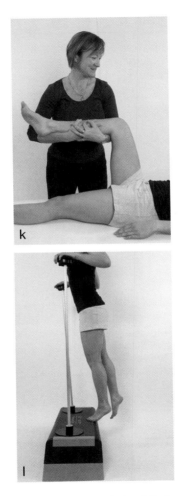

Fig 2.39—cont'd (k) resisted knee flexion (L5), (l) resisted ankle plantarflexion in weight-bearing (S1).

Nerve root pain

Once non-musculoskeletal causes for an athlete's symptoms have been ruled out, the next stage of the triaging process is to determine any nerve root involvement. The existence of nerve root pathology is not necessarily cause for alarm, but due to the possibility of an irreversible loss of motor or sensory function, all nerve root symptoms and signs must be closely monitored and referred for further investigations and opinion if a lack of improvement is not noted within about a month, depending on the severity of changes.

Pattern recognition in low back pain

Good use of subjective questioning and a thorough physical examination should aid you as a clinician in identifying specific common clinical conditions. Some fundamental principles include:

- Differentiating between involvement of radicular (neural – nerve root/peripheral nerve) and somatic (non-neural – discs/joints/muscle) structures

  - Radicular pain is usually more severe in its quality and is often described as "horrible or nasty" pain as opposed to the "dull ache" of somatic symptoms
  - Symptoms are usually more severe distally with unilateral leg or hand pain – worse than back or neck pain
  - The distribution of pain is linear — travels or shoots down the limb – either along the dermatome or peripheral nerve path
  - Pain is often associated with paraesthesia or anaesthesia (BUT not necessarily)
  - Motor weakness and reduced reflex responses may be present
  - Neural provocation tests are positive. **NB:** In cases of chronic or minor nerve irritation (that often mimic other musculoskeletal conditions), the patient's symptoms may be more subtle in quality and may not be associated with any neck or back pain. In these instances, the most significant findings are often the neural provocation tests. E.g. straight leg raise (SLR) (Fig 2.40)

2

Assessment and diagnosis of the injured athlete

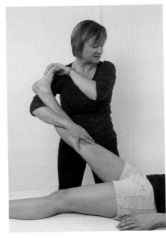

Fig 2.40   Straight leg raise test for neural provocation of the sciatic nerve and branches.

Minor nerve irritations and the "sports injuries" they mimic

Tennis elbow – radial nerve/posterior interosseous nerve (see Fig 2.11)
Golfer's elbow – ulnar nerve (see Fig 2.12)
DeQuervains tenosynovitis – radial nerve (see Fig 2.11)
Hamstring strain – sciatic nerve (see Figs 2.40 & 2.22)
Patellofemoral pain syndrome – femoral nerve
Shin splints/compartment syndromes – tibial/common peroneal nerve
Lateral ankle sprain – common peroneal nerve
Achilles tendinopathy – tibial nerve
Plantar fasciitis – calcaneal nerve/plantar nerves

- Identifying the involved level
- Confirming a nociceptive pain behaviour if a somatic structure is affected
  - Nociceptive pain tends to be fairly easy for the patient to localize in its distribution. Referred pain is often present, but this is specific in its location and quality

– The symptoms have a predictable and consistent response to movement and generally respond to painkillers and NSAIDs
• Determining an inflammatory/ischaemic or mechanical source of pain

All nociceptive pain is caused by one of these three sources stimulating pain fibres in the periphery. Identification of the source of pain will help determine the most appropriate management strategies to be used.

Physical examination

Most common clinical patterns have a predictable response to movement and testing. Key elements of the examination include:

Observation: Is there an obvious deformity/shift/protective posture? Is it correctable and what happens to the patient's symptoms when you do so?

Active movements: Does the movement occur evenly at all levels? Does the patient deviate from a symmetrical path? Range/quality and response should all be assessed

Combined movements: Specifically load certain areas of the motion segment to determine structures affected and guide treatment progression (Fig 2.41)

Sustained and repeated movements: Examine the effect of creep on spinal structures. Certain structures – discs/ligaments – are more prone to the effect of creep

Adjacent joints: The influence of shoulder and hip movement on the biomechanics of the adjacent spinal regions should not be underestimated and must be examined even when no pain exists at a distance away from the spinal structures

Neurological examination: Sensation, muscle power and reflexes

Neural provocation tests: It is essential that these are done accurately and with great sensitivity in order to identify subtle irritations of the neural structures

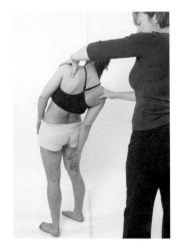

Fig 2.41 Lumbar quadrant demonstrating the combined movements of extension, lateral flexion and rotation.

Manual examination: Passive physiological intervertebral movements (PPIVMs) and passive accessory intervertebral movements (PAIVMs) are manual examination techniques performed by the clinician. Both help determine the relative mobility of the spinal region by identifying areas of segmental spinal hypermobility where there is greater movement between two adjacent spinal segments (e.g. L4 and L5), and areas of hypomobility in which movement between two adjacent spinal segments is reduced. The movements tested are either physiological movements – flexion/extension/lateral flexion and rotation, or accessory movements – along the planes of the vertebral bodies or the facet joints. These motion tests also identify pain provoking segments, both locally and referred. Manual examination should also include assessment of soft tissue changes and muscle tone in the region.

Yellow flags in the athletic population

We tend to associate the presence of psychological risk factors for the development of long-term disability or distress or "yellow flags", with inactive, poorly motivated patients. Yet, our athletic population is equally vulnerable to the effects of these psychosocial factors as pain and injury can have a large impact on their sporting careers, trust in their body and confidence in future performance. Believing that pain and activity are damaging, the adoption of a sick role and low mood as a result of injury are all risk factors associated with the development of chronic problems to which the athlete may succumb. Athletes are also highly vulnerable to the influence of conflicting advice and suggestions of a "fix or cure" for ongoing problems. It is not at all uncommon for them to have seen numerous clinicians, many promising a solution to their problem. This maintains the belief that something is structurally wrong and must be "fixed".

We owe it to all our patients to ensure that we explain both the structural pathology and pain physiology of their condition, as well as identify any athletes who may be "at risk" or exhibiting "yellow flags" and direct them towards appropriate intervention. The reader is referred to the noigroup website (www.noigroup.com) for excellent courses on the subject of pain physiology and pain management as well as a clinical forum and clinical information that can help develop expertise in this area.

At the end of the examination, you should clearly have identified:

- The presence of serious pathology
- Non-spinal problems
- Nerve root or neurological deficits
- Spinal pathology with a common clinical pattern.

These will be discussed in more detail in the following sections.

2

Assessment and diagnosis of the injured athlete

Common Injuries in the Spine

Disc Injuries

Lumbar disc prolapse

Disc problems can range from small minor irritations associated with tears of the annulus to frank protrusions of nuclear material into the spinal canal. Symptoms usually, but not always, correlate with the extent of the pathology. Discal injures are common in sports involving prolonged periods of flexion including cycling and rowing as well as sports with large rotational components such as golf.

Subjective:

Unilateral low back pain with referred pain into the posterior leg (dull, aching quality) ✓✓
Pain with lumbar flexion and sitting ✓✓✓
Pain increased with sustained flexion ✓✓✓
Pain aggravated by coughing and sneezing ✓✓

Objective:

Antalgic posture – spinal flexion and associated pelvic shift ✓✓
Limited forward flexion with increased area of symptoms ✓✓
Increased symptoms with sustained flexion and difficulty returning to a neutral position ✓✓

Special tests:

Positive straight leg raise (reduced range and pain increased by sensitizing manoeuvres, e.g. ankle dorsiflexion/hip adduction) ✓✓✓ (see Fig 2.40)
Symptoms centralize with repeated lumbar extension ✓✓

Associated injury:

Nerve root irritation is commonly associated with a disc prolapse. If nerve root irritation is present, pain is more severe in quality, extends further into the distal limb and is more severe in this region. Low back pain is often absent

Management:

Manual mobilization – lumbar rotation techniques very useful

McKenzie repeated extension exercises (Fig 2.42)

Neural mobilizing techniques

Avoidance of sitting and lumbar flexion – encourage standing, walking and lying down

Cervical disc injuries

Depending on the duration of symptoms, cervical disc injuries result in a wide range of clinical signs and symptoms. Traumatic injuries, such as those sustained on the rugby pitch or in gymnastics may result in a rapid onset of symptoms, while athletes participating in sports involving sustained activities such as rowing may have a history of minor neck problems that ultimately leads to more severe pathology.

Subjective:

Cloward's areas (Fig 2.43) – "clumps" of pain along the medial border of the scapula ✓✓✓

Specific region of pain difficult for patient to localize, but more severe in intensity than neck pain ✓✓

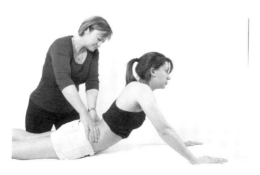

Fig 2.42 McKenzie repeated extension exercise.

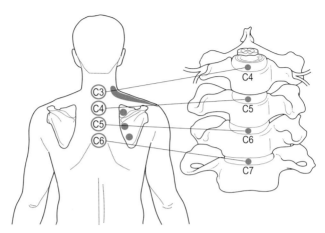

Fig 2.43 Discogenic pain referred from the lower cervical discs. Adapted from Maitland – *Vertebral Manipulation 7e*, with permission.

Neck stiffness and restricted mobility ✓✓

Pain increased with sustained flexion ✓

Cloward RB (1959) Cervical discography: A contribution to the etiology and mechanism of neck, shoulder and arm pain. Annals of Surgery 150:1052-1064

Objective:

Poke chin posture with increased scapular protraction ✓✓

Pain in Cloward's areas reproduced with cervical movements – rotation and cervical manual segmental examination ✓✓✓

Movement restriction variable, but usually some restriction to flexion and rotation ✓✓

"Trigger points" present in regions of Cloward's areas – painful to palpate with increased muscle tone ✓✓

Central and unilateral segmental hypomobility and tenderness ✓✓✓

Positive neural provocation test ✓

Management:

Manual mobilization

Neural mobilizing techniques

Specific postural re-education and motor control retraining

Thoracic disc injuries

Rare – due to inherently stable nature of the thoracic region and rib cage

Symptoms of pain and stiffness centrally in spinal region – may radiate "through the chest"

May be associated with thoracic nerve irritation – pain radiating around the chest wall

Upper thoracic disc injuries – may have associated sympathetic factors

Nerve root injury

Lumbar nerve root irritation

One of the most painful spinal conditions that ironically often presents with an absence of spinal pain. For this reason it is often misdiagnosed by clinicians, especially if neurological changes are also absent.

Subjective:

Severe and distressing unilateral limb pain often with associated pins and needles/ numbness ✓✓✓

Difficulty sleeping ✓✓

Absence of back pain ✓✓✓

Pain follows a dermatomal pattern within the limb (see Fig 2.38) – often worse in the distal dermatome. NB: may present with pain in the distal dermatome **ONLY** ✓✓✓

Pain increased by movements that reduce the size of the intervertebral foramen (extension/ipsilateral lateral flexion and rotation) ✓✓

Objective:

Patient looks unwell

Antalgic posture – reduced weight-bearing of the lower limb ✓✓

Symptoms aggravated by spinal extension and lateral flexion ✓✓✓

Pain increased by movements that tension the nerve tissue – positive neural provocation tests ✓✓✓

Neurological changes ✓

NSAIDs/simple analgesics – little help ✓✓

Special tests:

Specific neurological examination essential to determine presence of any compromise of the system and monitor improvement

Vibration testing for minor nerve compromise (Fig 2.44)

Associated features:

Individual anatomical variations may make patients more vulnerable to neural compromise, e.g. small spinal canal

Management:

Advice regarding positions of ease/activity modification

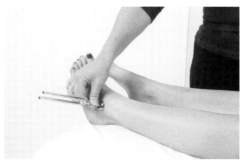

Fig 2.44 Testing for altered vibration sensitivity in patients with suspected nerve root irritation.

Manual techniques to open intervertebral foramen
Neural mobilizing techniques to encourage axoplasmic flow

Cervical nerve root irritation

Cervical nerve root injuries are one of the nastiest problems that patients can experience. Neuropathic pain is often most severe at night and disrupts sleep with patients expressing difficulty finding a position of comfort. Nerve root irritation is commonly associated with disc injury, especially in cases of trauma in younger athletes with higher water content in their discs.

Subjective:

Severe upper limb pain ± pins and needles/numbness in a dermatomal distribution ✓✓✓ (see Fig 2.38)

Upper limb symptoms more severe than neck symptoms ✓✓✓

Neck stiffness and restricted mobility ✓✓

Pain increased with movements that "close down" the facet joints on the affected side (extension/lateral flexion and rotation towards the side of symptoms) or "tension" the neural tissue (flexion and lateral flexion away from the side of symptoms) ✓✓✓

Objective:

Looks unwell and assumes a protective posture – unloading the neural structures and opening up the joints on the affected side ✓✓

Cervical movements are extremely restrictive and very provocative of the patient's symptoms ✓✓✓

Positive neurological signs ✓

Positive ULNPTs ✓✓✓ (see Figs 2.9, 2.11, 2.12)

Unilateral segmental hypomobility and tenderness at a level comparable with the dermatomal distribution of symptoms ✓✓✓

Management:

Advice regarding sleeping posture and positions of ease – reducing "tension" on the neural structures

Assessment and diagnosis of the injured athlete

2

Ensure adequate pain relief – may benefit from drugs for neuropathic pain

Manual mobilization – to open the joint on the affected side. Side glide and rotation techniques often very effective

Gentle neural mobilizing techniques

Specific postural re-education and motor control retraining

"Stingers"

A slang term for the transient neuropraxia often seen in contact sports such as rugby. The symptoms may arise from traction to the brachial plexus or nerve root, compression of the nerve root by the cervical spine or a direct blow to the brachial plexus.

Subjective:

Transient upper limb burning type pain ✓✓✓

Associated pins and needles and a sensation of weakness ✓✓✓

Players describe their arm as feeling "dead" or "numb" ✓✓✓

Objective:

Full cervical range of motion ✓✓✓

Full shoulder range of motion ✓✓✓

Normal ULNPTs ✓✓✓

Normal neurological testing ✓✓✓

Investigations:

These are not generally required unless symptoms worsen, persist or the player experiences recurrent problems

If the injury involves widespread neck pain or extensive symptoms in the limbs, further investigations are also warranted

Management:

As symptoms are usually transient, treatment is often not required. Players should be monitored for altered or persistent symptoms that may require specific management

Bony injuries

Pars interarticularis stress fracture

This is one of the most common injuries in athletes whose sports involve high levels of lumbar hyperextension such as gymnasts, cricketers, high jumpers and divers. Athletes are usually in their teens/early 20s, where immature bone is placed under excessive levels of strain.

Subjective:

Unilateral low back pain with activity (dull, aching quality) ✓✓✓

Referred pain – posterior thigh to knee ✓

Symptoms may progress to pain at rest and at night

Objective:

Active and passive extension ± ipsilateral lateral flexion – pain ✓✓✓

Excessive movement at one vertebral level – into extension (hinging) ✓

Tight hamstrings ✓✓

Palpation – tender over involved vertebral segment ✓✓

Investigations:

CT imaging (Fig 2.45) — high levels of radiation

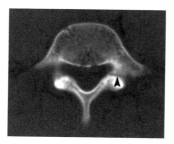

Fig 2.45   CT image showing a pars defect.

2

Assessment and diagnosis of the injured athlete

Special test:

Lumbar quadrant ± one leg standing ✓✓ (Figs 2.41 and 2.46)

Associated injury:

Development of spondylolisthesis – bilateral symptoms
May have associated neurological signs – pins and needles

Management: (see also Case Study in Section 3 p 230)

Symptom driven treatment. Evidence suggests that there is no correlation between a patient's symptoms and the associated imaging

Avoidance of aggravating activities – running/jumping

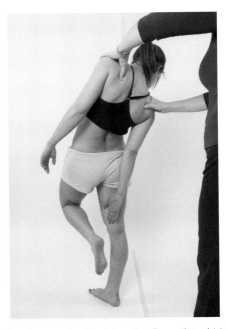

Fig 2.46 Lumbar quadrant in 1 leg standing – thought to increase the compression through the affected spinal region.

Normalize movement patterns

Emphasis on gluteal activation and hip extension, spinal control and hamstring length (see Figs 2.23 and 3.26)

Spondylolisthesis

This condition describes the anterior displacement of a vertebra or the vertebral column in relation to the vertebrae below. It may be congenital (isthmic) or develop secondary to bilateral pars stress fractures. Therefore it is associated with similar sports and activities to those resulting in pars stress fractures such as cricket or gymnastics.

Subjective:

Bilateral low back pain with somatic referred pain into the proximal limbs ✓✓✓

Radicular symptoms – pain/pins and needles/numbness in the lower limbs ✓

Pain increased by extension activities ✓✓✓

Catches of pain associated with normal daily activities ✓✓

Episodes of intermittent back spasms ✓✓

Objective:

Tenderness on palpation of involved level ✓✓✓

Overactive erector spinae/stiff spine ✓✓✓

Tight hamstrings ✓✓✓

Investigations:

Imaging – slip visible on lateral X-ray view

Special tests:

Shear test – increased translation of one vertebral level of the level above (Fig 2.47)

Management:

Specific spinal stabilizing exercises (O'Sullivan et al 1997) Hamstring stretches

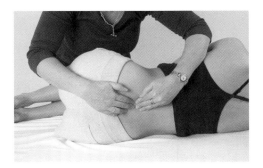

Fig 2.47 Shear test.

  Hip extension mobilization and gluteal strengthening
O'Sullivan PB, Twomey LT and Allison GT (1997) Evaluation of specific stabilizing exercise in the treatment of chronic low back pain with radiologic diagnosis of spondylolysis or spondylolisthesis. Spine 22:2959-2967

Spinal joint problems

Lumbar zygapophyseal (facet) joint irritation

Irritation of the zygapophyseal joints is often associated with degenerative changes in the spine. Individual joint involvement is common with extension overload of the joint, however, in cases of degenerative changes, bilateral and multi-level symptoms and signs are more usual. The extent of the symptoms and signs is usually comparable with the extent of the pathology.

Subjective:

Unilateral low back pain ± somatic referred pain into the proximal limbs (dull, aching quality) ✓✓✓
Referred pain rarely extends below the knee ✓✓✓
Pain with extension related activities – walking and standing, especially prolonged ✓✓✓

NB: people who sit in "active extension" with overactivity of the erector spinae and an increased lumbar lordosis. Sitting is normally associated with lumbar flexion and would therefore normally be expected to reduce pain in patient's with spondylolisthesis, but if a patient sits in "active extension", this activity may be painful. (O'Sullivan 2005) (Fig 2.48)

O'Sullivan P (2005) Diagnosis and classification of chronic low back pain disorders: maladaptive movement and motor control impairments as underlying mechanism. Manual Therapy 10:242-255

Objective:

Pain reproduced with movements that close the facet joint down ✓✓✓

Tenderness on unilateral manual segmental examination of the joint ✓✓✓

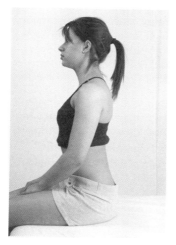

Fig 2.48   Active extension movement pattern.

Pain may be alleviated by opening techniques – but not always as these positions may stretch an inflamed joint capsule and surrounding ligamentous structures

Special tests:

Quadrant – combined position of extension/lateral flexion / rotation – close packed position of the facet joint

Management:

Postural correction – reduce lordosis – improve abdominal strength

Manual mobilization techniques to improve joint nutrition and encourage blood flow

Mobilizing exercises – into positions of ease

Cervical zygapophyseal (facet) joint injuries

The most frequent cervical injuries in athletes are probably acute strains and sprains of the soft tissue structures of the neck. These involve the ligamentous and capsular structures of the cervical joints and it is often difficult to differentiate the specific structures involved. Sporting accidents are the second most common cause, after road traffic accidents, of acute neck injuries with a high incidence of recurrence following an initial injury. Older athletes usually have some associated degenerative changes in the region, mostly at C5–7, making the development of symptoms more common.

Subjective:

Traumatic injury or may be associated with sustained/ repetitive activities

Gradual onset of worsening symptoms

Unilateral neck pain of a dull aching quality – localized to the involved segment and 1-2 segments above and/or below due to the innervation of the facet joint and related structures ✓✓✓

Referred pain over trapezius region extending to the deltoid area – depending on segment involved ✓✓

Painfully restricted movement towards the side of pain – rotation/lateral flexion ✓✓✓

Pain on elevation of the upper limb ✓

Objective:

Restricted mobility – unilateral with mechanical behaviour ✓✓✓

Closing down pattern – extension/lateral flexion/rotation ✓✓✓

PAIVM's – hypomobile and tender unilaterally ✓✓✓

Positive ULNPTs if IVF narrowed/inflammation present ✓ (see Figs 2.9, 2.11, 2.12)

Management:

PRICE – if acute

Manual mobilization

Soft tissue work

Active exercise programme – mobility exercises and specific control exercises to prevent recurrence

Neural mobilizing techniques if appropriate

Headaches of musculoskeletal origin

A musculoskeletal cause of headaches in an athlete is one of several hundred possible diagnoses. It is essential for the clinician to eliminate other causes of headaches including those relating to hydration/nutrition and metabolic causes, often requiring involvement of a physician in the patient's management. Two common headaches of musculoskeletal origin are tension headaches and cervicogenic headaches related to the neck joints. It is worth remembering that although there are certain criteria and characteristics for various headaches, an individual may present with features of more than one type.

Subjective:

Tension headaches

Symptoms are described as a tight band across the forehead. It is pressing although not pulsating ✓✓

Bilateral symptoms that are mild to moderate in intensity ✓✓✓

Duration −30 minutes to several days

Associated symptoms are rare (nausea/photophobia)

Rarely aggravated by physical activity

Cervicogenic headaches

Unilateral moderate to severe symptoms associated with ipsilateral neck pain ✓✓✓

Symptoms originate in the cervical spine and the onset of the headache can be associated with the development of neck pain ✓✓✓

Associated presence of upper limb pain and symptoms ✓

Frequency is more variable than with other forms of headaches

Associated with prolonged postures, movements of the head or any physical activity which may increase the load and stress placed on the joints ✓✓✓

Objective:

Tension headaches

Subtle end range restrictions to movement – flexion/lateral flexion/rotation but no reproduction of headache ✓✓

Palpable trigger points in several muscle groups with reproduction of athlete's symptoms ✓✓✓ (Fig 2.49)

Cervicogenic headaches

Restricted range of neck motion ✓✓✓

Hypomobility in one or more segments of the upper cervical spine – unilateral and comparable with the side of the headache ✓✓✓

Reproduction of athlete's symptoms on manual examination of the cervical spine ✓

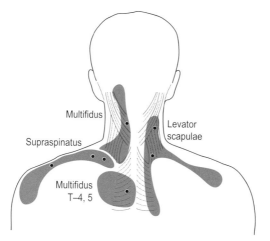

Fig 2.49 Sites of trigger point referral from muscles commonly producing tension headaches. Reproduced by permission of www.headache.com.au.

Management:

Manual therapy – mobilization ± manipulation

Soft tissue release work – beneficial in reducing the tightness and tension in the muscles of the back, shoulders and neck

Dry needling/IMS – trigger point therapy

Strengthening exercises for the postural muscles of the neck and shoulders may also be beneficial by reducing the tension held in other muscles and providing more support for the head and neck in upright positions

Relaxation and stress relieving techniques

Ergonomic and postural advice relating to sport and general daily living

Sports related whiplash

Whiplash is a term more frequently associated with motor vehicle accidents, however the high forces involved in many contact sports or the accidents sustained in activities such as skiing or equestrian pursuits often lead to athletes presenting with signs and symptoms similar to whiplash associated disorder (WAD)

Subjective:

Multi-factorial aetiology – patients can therefore present with a wide range of symptoms and signs ✓✓✓

May not report symptoms at time of incident

Spread of symptoms common

Non-dermatomal distribution due to widespread pathology

Bizarre descriptions of pain – sympathetic involvement

Variable response to analgesia

Neck pain ✓✓

Neck stiffness ✓✓

Upper limb pain ± paraesthesia ✓

Headaches ✓✓✓

Problems with memory/concentration

Visual disturbances

Psychological distress ✓

Recognise that a so-called "whiplash profile" has been described in which patients presenting with WAD have higher scores for psychological factors including somatization, depression and obsessive-compulsive behaviour

Objective:

Investigations: X-ray/MRI findings NAD ✓✓ however it is suspected by many experts that microtrauma (not visible on X-Ray or MRI) is present. This may include:

- Bone bruising/oedema
- Microfractures
- Disc lesions/contusions
- Ligamentous injury
- Muscular damage
- Neural irritation

Significant irritability ✓✓

Reduced and painful cervical range of motion – variable and multidirectional ✓✓

Presence of muscular spasm

Gross neurological examination normal

Examination of vibration sensitivity positive (see Fig 2.44)

Positive upper limb neural provocation testing (I, IIa/b, III) ✓✓ (Figs 2.9, 2.11, 2.12)

Evidence of hyperalgesia and allodynia– heightened response to sensory input – evidence of central sensitization ✓

NB: check stability of upper cervical spine

Management:

Active movement – advice to keep active

Specific motor control exercises

Neural mobilizing techniques (specific to assessment findings)

Correction of scapular position and control

Correction of cervical posture and control

Psychological input ✓

Thoracic spine and rib injuries

Thoracic spine wedge fracture

Compression fractures in young athletes are rare, but may be associated with traumatic injuries such as falls from a horse or a height (gymnastics). It is important to consider eating disorders or underlying pathology (osteoporosis/cancer/tumours) in all cases that may predispose individuals to spinal fractures.

Subjective:

Constant, unremitting pain ✓✓✓

Associated irritation/compression of the spinal cord – paraesthesia/anaesthesia – upper/lower limbs ✓

Objective:

Exquisite tenderness over the involved vertebral level ✓✓✓

Investigations:

Confirmed on X-ray/CT scan ✓✓✓

Bone scan – in non-traumatic cases – determine age of fracture

Management:

Stable fracture – therefore no need for surgical intervention

Pain medication

Activity modification

Specific exercise therapy – facilitate thoracic multifidus activation

   – scapular stabilizers/retractors
   – spinal extensors

Thoracic outlet syndrome

This condition is a collection of symptoms resulting from compromise of the neural and vascular structures passing through the thoracic outlet between the clavicle, first rib and scalene muscles. Symptoms may arise from either compression or stretch of the brachial plexus, subclavian artery and/or vein. Patients can present with a range of symptoms, depending on the extent of the compromise and which structures are most affected. The cause of the compromise is often associated with repetitive postures and activities, and therefore is often seen in the sporting population.

Subjective:

Neurological

Pain in the upper limb especially at night or on waking ✓✓✓

Pins and needles/numbness in fingers and hands ✓

Clumsiness and uncoordinated movements ✓

Vascular

Cramping pain in hands and fingers ✓
Discoloration – circulatory changes ✓✓
Sensations of heaviness in hand and upper limb ✓✓✓
Feelings of swelling/puffiness in hand ✓

Objective:

Forward head posture with overactive scalenes/
sternocleidomastoid (SCM) ✓
Altered scapulae position – protracted/retracted or
downwardly rotated ✓✓✓
Hypomobility low cervical/upper thoracic joints ✓✓✓
Hypomobile 1st rib ✓✓
Positive ULNPTs 1 (median) and/or 3 (ulnar) ✓✓✓
(see Figs 2.9 and 2.12)
Objective numbness/muscle weakness

Investigations:

X-ray – if the presence of a cervical rib is suspected

Special tests:

These provocative tests aim to compromise the neural and
vascular structures using extreme postures of the upper
limb and neck in association with circulatory demand. Look
for a reproduction of the patient's symptoms, but also
examine for changes in limb colour and swelling

Adson's test

• Extension and rotation of cervical spine with deep
  inspiration
• Obliterates radial pulse
• 20% asymptomatics positive

Abd/ER test

• Shoulders positioned at 90° Abd/ER
• Squeezing hands should reproduce symptoms

2

Assessment and diagnosis of the injured athlete

Sustained shoulder girdle elevation/depression

May reproduce symptoms

May be evidence of a Horner's syndrome

Management:

Patient specific management to address the relevant postural deformities contributing to the patient's symptoms

Joint mobilization – cervical/thoracic spine/ribs

Soft tissue release – scalenes/pectorals/levator scapulae

Motor control re-education – scapulae/cervical spine

Scheuermann's disease

This disease affects adolescents and is thought to be a form of spinal osteochondrosis. Osteochondrosis is a disease characterized by interruption of the blood supply of a bone, in particular to the epiphyses. In Scheuermann's disease this results in the vertebrae developing in a wedge shape, as the anterior aspect of the vertebral bodies ceases to grow during adolescence, while the posterior aspect continues to develop. It most commonly occurs in the thoracic spine, leading to a significant increase in the thoracic kyphosis.

Subjective:

Patients are usually males and present with symptoms towards the end of their growth spurt ✓✓✓

Pain is localized to the spinal region, primarily the apex of the thoracic kyphosis ✓✓✓

Associated symptoms of pain and stiffness in other spinal regions and limbs can occur due to adverse neural pathodynamics associated with the spinal deformity ✓✓

Symptoms are often aggravated by physical activity and by long periods of standing or sitting ✓✓✓

Objective:

Increased thoracic kyphosis that cannot be corrected actively by the patient and remains present in both prone and supine lying ✓✓✓

Generalized hypomobility in the thoracic spine – PPIVMs and PAIVMs ✓✓✓

Investigations:

X-ray imaging demonstrates wedge shaped thoracic vertebrae, often with herniated discs and Schmorl's nodes (protrusions of the discs through the vertebral end plates)

Associated injury:

This condition is not a disease and does not "spread"; however it is common for other structures to be affected by the structural deformity. Increased strain is placed on both the cervical and lumbar regions to compensate for the deformity and surrounding soft tissues become restricted (pectorals/erector spinae). Pain may develop from these structures or the neural structures as mentioned previously

Management:

Active exercise is essential to maintain spinal mobility and prevent secondary problems developing from the neural structures and soft tissue

A good programme focused on scapular control, thoracic extension and abdominal activation will help support the structural deformity

Hydrotherapy

T4 syndrome

As the name syndrome suggests, T4 syndrome is a collection of symptoms rather than a specific disease. It is characterized by pain and paraesthesia in the upper arms ± neck and back pain. Diagnosis is usually by exclusion as many other disorders reproduce similar symptoms and signs. Athletes experiencing this problem are often involved in sporting activities with prolonged or excessive periods of thoracic flexion.

Subjective:

Pain in the upper limb extending to the hand ± paraesthesia ✓✓✓

Unilateral/bilateral "glove" distribution of paraesthesia to the hands ✓✓✓

Pain in the head, neck and upper thoracic region ✓✓

Symptoms described as heaviness/"nerve type"/cramping (possibly reflective of involvement of the sympathetic nervous system) ✓✓

Objective:

Symptoms reproduced with cervical movements ✓✓✓

Symptoms reproduced ± alleviated by mobilization/ manipulation of the upper thoracic segments (often T4) ✓✓✓

Positive upper limb neural provocation testing (I, IIa/b, III) ✓✓✓ (see Figs 2.9, 2.11, 2.12)

Differential diagnosis:

Cervical/upper thoracic dysfunction

Thoracic outlet syndrome

Cardiac disease

Neurological disease

Spinal tumour/metastasis

Management:

Manual therapy – mobilization ± manipulation

Soft tissue release work

Neural mobilizing techniques (specific to assessment findings)

Correction of scapular position and control

Correction of cervical posture and control

Costovertebral joint sprain

A condition commonly seen in athletes involved in throwing or overhead activities.

Subjective:

Patients often appear very disabled by the pain resulting from a costovertebral (CV) joint sprain as any body movement places stress on the region ✓✓✓

Localized sharp pain over the CV joint with aching pain in the surrounding region ✓✓✓

Pain is constant and intense, associated with CV joint movement as a result of respiration. Pain increased by deep breathing and coughing ✓✓✓

Pain increased by arm elevation and thoracic movements ✓✓

Objective:

Reduced depth of respiration ✓✓✓

Splinting of the trunk and rib cage to avoid movement of the ribs ✓✓✓

Symptoms aggravated by thoracic rotation and lateral flexion – both towards and away from the side of symptoms ✓✓✓

Tenderness on specific palpation of the CV joint (but rarely associated with hypermobility; manual segmental examination more commonly demonstrates hypomobility due to protective splinting) ✓✓✓

Management:

PRICE

Scapular taping to support the injured joint region

Scapular retraction exercises to enhance support for the injured region

Rib fractures

Traumatic rib fractures are frequent in all sports, involving either a blow to the chest or a fall, and as such are

2

Assessment and diagnosis of the injured athlete

reasonably easy to diagnose. More commonly mis-diagnosed are stress fractures. These usually occur in the 5th to 9th ribs at areas of muscular insertion for muscles such as serratus anterior, latissimus dorsi, pectoralis major and the external obliques. Stress fractures often occur in golfers, rowers and gymnasts.

Subjective:

Traumatic injury or history of intensive training/activity ✓✓✓

Chest pain over the rib region ✓✓✓

Patient experiences difficulty breathing and pain associated with deep breathing ✓✓✓

Painful thoracic and arm movements – flexion/abduction ✓✓✓

Restricted mobility ✓

Objective:

Constant pain localized to the involved rib/s with little referred pain ✓✓✓

Night pain ✓

Pain with deep breathing/coughing ✓✓✓

Muscle spasm (may produce referral) ✓✓

Differential diagnosis:

Specific palpation of the painful region in chest wall is essential in establishing a diagnosis

No palpable crepitus or clicking with stress fractures

Stress fractures – no pain with rib springing away from the site of injury (Fig 2.50)

It is important to differentiate between a strain of the intercostals and a bony injury with specific palpation of the intercostal muscles and along the line of the rib

Management:

Appropriate pain relief and rest

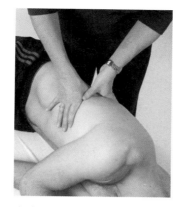

Fig 2.50 Rib springing to detect presence of a stress fracture.

Encourage deep breathing and maintenance of movement
Review of technique in the case of stress fractures

Things to note:

With any traumatic injury, it is important to consider the
possibility of internal organ damage
It is essential to ensure that the history of the injury is
compatible with the extent of the injury – consideration
must always be given to the effect of amenorrhea in female
athletes, as well as the possible existence of tumours or
bony secondaries

Intercostal muscle strain

These small muscles are commonly strained during sporting
activities that involve vigorous or excessive movements of
the upper limbs or trunk. Sports that may cause this type of
injury include golf and tennis. They can also occur as a result
of unaccustomed activity, such as a return to heavy training
after a period of rest or deconditioning.

Subjective:

Dull aching pain in the lateral chest region ✓✓✓

Pain exacerbated by deep breathing and coughing ✓✓✓

Pain exacerbated by thoracic spine movements and/or arm movements ✓✓✓

Objective:

Pain on palpation of the intercostal muscles ✓✓✓

Pain exacerbated by thoracic spine movements and/or arm movements ✓✓✓. The specific aggravating movements are patient specific and often relate to the incident or activity of onset

Differential diagnosis:

These muscles can be strained with similar movements and activities to those that may result in stress fractures of the ribs. It is therefore essential to palpate the region accurately to determine if the area of tenderness is localized to the rib or the muscle between two ribs. While management is similar in both cases, differences exist in terms of providing the athlete with an accurate prognosis and advice regarding return to play

Management:

Ensure adequate pain relief

Ice (in the initial 48 hours) or heat (may provide greater comfort and pain relief to the patient)

Advice regarding deep breathing exercises and supported coughing

Encourage active movement of the upper limbs and trunk within the limits of pain

Treatment and Rehabilitation

SECTION

3

Introduction

All rehabilitation programmes utilized by physiotherapists must be **goal driven**, but nowhere is this more important than in sports and exercise medicine, where athletes are commonly focused on one specific event. Textbooks and the internet abound with treatment recipes and ladders for the rehabilitation of specific conditions. While these can serve as a useful starting point, rehabilitation programmes must be designed for each individual athlete, as every injury is different and athletes' body types, sporting demands and timeframes for return to sport will be very different.

The use of patient-specific goals, decided together with the individual athlete, will help formulate a programme using clinical reasoning to determine effective and time-appropriate treatment modalities.

Involving the athlete in the programme design also helps to engage them in the process and keep them motivated. Rehabilitation episodes can be frustrating, worrying and sometimes even depressing periods for athletes. A good clinician ensures that the athlete (and they themselves) remains interested and engaged by ensuring that the programme is focused, relevant and varied. Positive programmes that focus on what the athlete *can* do are more likely to be complied with than programmes that emphasize the negative and focus on what they *can't do*.

The previous section dealt with assessment of the injured athlete. This is necessary to diagnose the athlete's condition and establish the athlete's reported problems, as well as identifying common findings usually associated with the pathology that must be considered when designing a rehabilitation programme.

Considering both the patient's reported problem and known features of the pathology will allow you to establish treatment goals. These goals are focused on the outcomes you are trying to achieve as a clinician.

When rehabilitating the athlete, common goals include:

- protecting the athlete from further injury
- controlling and reducing pain and swelling
- restoring full and pain free movement to the injured area
- normalizing motor control and movement patterns, e.g. gait re-education in the lower limb, scapulo-humeral rhythm in the upper limb
- establishing effective trunk control and proximal stability for limb function
- restoring the strength, endurance and power of the injured area sufficient to allow safe and effective return to play
- restoring any proprioceptive deficits
- preventing re-injury by addressing any relevant extrinsic and intrinsic factors, e.g. equipment, biomechanics

Once established, these treatment goals will determine the **physiological processes** of the patient's system that you need to affect (stimulate and / or inhibit) in order to achieve the required clinical effect. These treatment goals are also based on the stage of tissue healing and pain mechanisms involved in the manifestation of the patient's symptoms. The reference below has a full explanation of pain mechanisms and the relationship with patient's symptoms.

Butler D (ed) (2000) The Sensitive Nervous System. Noigroup Publications, Adelaide, Australia.

This is an essential stage of the clinical reasoning process as it provides the rationale behind the use of all treatment modalities including:

- Manual therapy – mobilization / manipulation / massage
- Exercise therapy – motor control / strength / endurance / power
- Taping and supports
- Electrophysical agents, e.g. TENS, ultrasound, interferential
- Acupuncture and dry needling
- Drug management and the use of injection therapy

Goals are generally divided into stages that facilitate progression of the rehabilitation programme. When

3

Treatment and Rehabilitation

considering stages of rehabilitation, the clinician needs to consider the pathophysiology of the injured and healing tissue, the existing signs and symptoms and how these relate to the stage of tissue healing and expected presentation, as well as the sporting requirements of the athlete. Criteria and assessment of return to play will be discussed in the next section.

Goals need to be reassessed regularly by reviewing the athlete's actual versus expected progress in order to ensure treatment effectiveness. If progress does not occur at the expected rate, both diagnosis and treatment need to be reviewed.

Errors in the rehabilitation process are most common in the initial, acute phase or in the final stages leading towards return to play. Some of the most common errors are listed in Box 3.1.

Box 3.1   Common errors in the rehabilitation process

Early stage

- Ongoing effusion – resulting in inhibition of muscle function and control
- Inadequate pain control – also causing poor muscle function
- Lack of isolated muscle activation – especially in the quadriceps and rotator cuff
- Use of compensatory muscle patterns – commonly seen in single leg stance and with arm elevation
- Loss of accessory joint motion limiting full range of motion

Late stage

- Lack of effusion control, especially in lower limb injuries where there is damage to joint surfaces
- Inadequate muscle strength
- Lack of focus on power component of rehabilitation
- Lack of sport specific drills – gap between clinical rehabilitation and return to training is too great

---

This section includes a number of case studies. These illustrate the goal driven focus of the rehabilitation process and are not designed to provide recipes for treatment. They also demonstrate the varying scenarios encountered in the field of sports and exercise medicine and the need for a multidisciplinary approach to player management.

Tissue healing

Tissue healing in most musculoskeletal injuries is generally a process of repair in which the damaged tissue is replaced by non-specific granulation tissue that eventually matures to form scar tissue.

Tim Watson has written extensively on the subject (www.electrotherapy.org). He divides the repair process into four stages and concludes that the repair process is a highly effective mechanism of tissue healing and the aim of all medical interventions should be to optimize, facilitate and support this process, rather than attempting to alter it in any capacity. Where extensive tissue damage has occurred, or in athletes where delayed responses have occurred, interventions may be appropriate to facilitate the normal process of repair, but no evidence exists to support any benefit in trying to change the body's own efficient processes.

When designing a rehabilitation programme, the clinician should consider the stage of tissue healing that is occurring during each phase of the rehabilitation process. Fig 3.1 illustrates the stages of tissue healing for "average tissue"

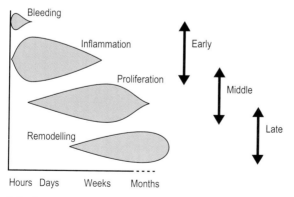

Fig 3.1 Stages of tissue healing and rehabilitation. Watson (2009) modified with permission.

3

Treatment and Rehabilitation

having sustained an "average injury" and the associated rehabilitation phases.

Bleeding phase

This happens following any tissue damage. The amount of bleeding depends on both the extent of the injury and the nature of the tissue damaged. Muscle tissue bleeds a lot and significant amounts of blood escapes within the tissues. Ligamentous tissue is far less vascularized which means there is very little bleeding. Average bleeding time is thought to be 6−8 hours post injury, but will also depend on the tissue damaged. Bleeding causes the release of various chemicals within the injured tissue which in turn stimulate the inflammatory cascade.

Inflammatory phase

Inflammation is not a bad thing. It is an essential part of the repair process because it ensures effective tissue healing. It starts within hours of the damage being sustained and in the average injury peaks at 2–3 days post injury. It then gradually subsides and concludes 2–3 weeks post injury. During the inflammatory phase, an exudate is produced that dilutes any toxins within the damaged area and forms the fibrin clot which acts as a barrier to foreign particles and debris. Certain cells released during this phase stimulate phagocytosis and tissue debridement. It is also the interaction of chemical mediators released by the inflammatory process that stimulates proliferation and ongoing repair. However, proper healing and repair require a well-regulated inflammatory response.

Occasionally, inflammation persists beyond the expected conclusion time or occurs in excess of the extent of tissue damage. Some of the reasons why a chronic inflammatory state may persist include contamination by foreign bodies or bacteria, invasion by microorganisms able to survive within large phagocytes, antigen–antibody reactions or continual irritation by mechanical stresses.

Proliferation phase

In this phase, starting 24–48 hours post injury, collagen material is produced that will form the scar tissue. This phase peaks at 2–3 weeks post injury, at which time the bulk of the scar material is produced that will eventually form the matured scar tissue. At the same time, angiogenesis (formation of new local blood vessels) occurs. This new blood flow provides nutrients and oxygen to the region, essential elements for collagen production. Both of these processes are stimulated by chemical mediators produced during the inflammatory phase. The proliferation phase continues until several months post injury, though in an ever declining role.

Remodelling phase

Scar tissue that is produced in the proliferation phase requires organizing to produce a scar that is capable of behaving in a similar way to the specific tissue it has replaced. The initial Type III collagen tissue is randomly orientated. In response to movement and stress, these tissues become orientated along the lines of stress, providing strength in specific, functional directions. At the same time, some of the Type III collagen is replaced with Type I collagen with more cross-links and greater tensile strength. This occurs during the remodelling phase which starts 1–2 weeks post injury, following the commencement of collagen production. It continues for several months post trauma, extending beyond the conclusion of the proliferation phase in order to produce a functional and organized scar.

Factors that may impede healing

- Excessive oedema
- Excessive bleeding and presence of haematoma
- Poor vascular supply
- Tissue separation
- Muscle spasm

3

Treatment and Rehabilitation

- Athlete's health, age, nutrition
- Use of corticosteroids / NSAIDs
- Presence of keloid / hypertrophic scars
- Presence of co-existing pathologies, e.g. diabetes
- Presence of infection
- Climate / temperature

PRICE

PRICE (Protection / Rest / Ice / Compression / Elevation) is the initial treatment modality of choice in the majority of sporting injuries. Use of the PRICE regime is thought to minimize pain and swelling and ensure a more rapid return to the playing field. As inflammation is a vital part of tissue healing and repair, it is essential to ensure that the use of a PRICE regime does not compromise this stage of the tissue healing process.

The following information is drawn from the evidence based guidelines produced by the Association of Chartered Physiotherapists in Sports Medicine (ACPSM) for the management of soft tissue injuries in the first 72 hours (www.acpsm.org). The latest version of these guidelines was published in November 2010.

P rotection

Protection ensures that no further tissue damage occurs and ensures that the fibrin network and collagen tissue are not disrupted.

For initial protection move the injured athlete from any location in which further injury may occur. In several sporting situations, such as the rugby field, sailing regatta, swimming pool or ice rink, this may be a far from straightforward exercise. It is essential that every clinician is familiar with procedures for retrieving people from the sporting environment of the competition. New clinicians should undergo an induction programme that familiarizes them with likely injury scenarios and the mechanisms for dealing with these.

Further protection may be provided in various ways. The use of this equipment will depend on the structure injured and the severity of the injury. Commonly used equipment includes:

- Crutches
- Slings
- Taping
- Bracing
- Splints

The nature and degree of protection will be based on the extent of the injury, the severity of pain experienced as well as the psychological profile of the athlete. Protection should be applied in the early stages post injury. Results from animal studies suggest that a moderate / Grade II injury requires 3–5 days to avoid excessive stress on healing tissues.

It is essential to ensure that the mode of protection or support is capable of accommodating any increase in oedema and that it does not totally immobilize the injured structure. Athletes need to be instructed to look for signs of excessive tightness and if these occur, to remove the bandage and contact the clinician.

Indications that bandages or splints are too tight include:

- Poor venous return in response to light finger pressure over a distal region. This is referred to as a blanching response. When a finger is gently pressed against healthy tissue (often over a finger nail), the underlying skin blanches or turns white. If blood flow to the region is normal, the tissue quickly returns to it's usual colour. The time taken for this to occur is called refill time. If blood flow is compromised, refill time is prolonged. The most effective way to determine this is to compare blanching responses and refill times between the bandaged and non bandaged limb.
- Swelling distal to the bandage or splint
- Feelings of pins and needles / numbness
- An increased level of pain

3

Treatment and Rehabilitation

Bandages and splints commonly become too tight at night when limbs are in dependent positions and a lack of normal mobility reduces venous return from limbs.

R est

Rest from aggravating activities is advocated in the early management of soft tissue injuries with a similar rationale to the use of protection. Previously, rest was prescribed until a return to pain-free activity was possible; however it is now recognized that some element of movement is essential to ensure scar tissue is laid down in an organized fashion that follows the lines of tissue strain. Research has shown that immobilization results in a disorganized orientation of scar tissue.

The concept of "relative rest" is considered more appropriate, especially in the athletic population who are likely to be resistant to the idea of total rest. In this case, controlled motion, within the limits of pain and avoiding undue stress on the healing tissue is permitted. The commencement of controlled movement will depend upon the grade of injury, anything from Day 1 for a minor Grade 1 injury to Day 5 for a severe Grade 3 condition.

I ce

Ice or Cryotherapy is thought to be useful in limiting the harmful effects of tissue damage. It should be recognized that although ice is widely used, research evidence regarding the physiological effects and the best methods of application is lacking. The general claims regarding the physiological effects of ice include lowering the temperature of the tissues, which results in vasoconstriction thus reducing excessive bleeding. Research evidence does not support a reduction in oedema, except when used in conjunction with compression and elevation. It is also proposed that ice causes a reduction in cellular metabolism which, together with vasoconstriction, limits the release of metabolic by-products and thereby reduces further cell death and tissue injury. Ice is also thought to reduce pain by slowing nerve conduction velocity and muscle spasm by reducing muscle spindle activity.

Although the research evidence is not conclusive, there is general agreement that the application of ice for 20–30 minutes every 2 hours is most effective in reducing pain, blood flow and metabolism. The best method of application is chipped or crushed ice, placed within a damp towel.

Clinical observation, again not supported by research evidence, suggests that care must be taken with the application of ice to avoid both superficial nerve damage and the production of an "ice burn". An ice burn occurs when skin is damaged from excessive exposure to low temperatures. Clinical signs of an "ice burn" include pain, swelling, redness and blistering of the skin. If ice is applied in an area of limited subcutaneous fat or over a superficial nerve, the recommended time is 10 minutes. In all cases, the skin condition and patient's pain response should be checked every 5 minutes.

C ompression

Compression also results in vasoconstriction and limitation of oedema. Restricting excessive inflammatory exudate results in a reduction of the inflammatory mediators that stimulate proliferation and ultimately scar tissue formation. Excessive oedema may become chronic, may limit range of motion or act to inhibit muscle function.

Several modes of compression are available including cheap and readily available elastic bandages (adhesive and non-adhesive), neoprene supports, inflatable splints and intermittent compression wraps.

Compression should always be applied in a distal to proximal direction ensuring uniform compression throughout. The area of compression should start at a reasonable distance below the level of the injury and extend to a reasonable distance above the injury. In the cases of peripheral limbs, this is usually to the joint above the injury.

3

Treatment and Rehabilitation

Compression structures must accommodate any increase in oedema. Immediately following application of the compressive material, distal circulation must be checked for signs of circulatory compromise and the athlete must be instructed on how to monitor for this on an ongoing basis (refer to section on Protection for further details).

Equally, compression bandages usually require reapplication within 24 hours to accommodate a resolution of swelling. In some cases, padding or gapping of the compressive material is needed to ensure adequate compression or relieve pressure on vulnerable areas. There is significant evidence to suggest that compression should be removed when the limb is elevated, but should be applied at all times when the limb is in a dependent position.

Acute ankle strapping

An inversion sprain of the ankle is one of the most common injuries that is strapped immediately post injury to control swelling and provide support.

Tape: 5 cm cohesive bandage or EAB (Elastic Adhesive Bandage)

> The Ankle is positioned as close to a neutral position as possible
>
> Use of a felt horseshoe around the lateral malleolus will prevent swelling from accumulating there (Fig 3.2a)

1. Starting medially above the toes, take the bandage laterally over the dorsum of the foot and encircle the distal aspect of the foot. Repeat the movement to lock the bandage in place.
2. Move proximally along the foot keeping the bandage overlapping by 50% to ensure even pressure.
3. At the level of the navicular bone, pass the bandage laterally over the heel and around the ankle in a figure of 8 movement, crossing the tape over directly above the anterior talo-fibular ligament (ATFL) or (Calcaneo-fibular ligament) CFL to provide additional support in the region of the damaged structure.

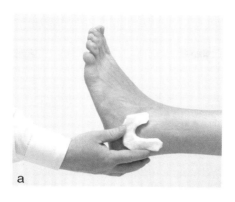

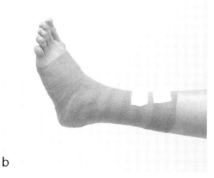

Fig 3.2 (a) A felt horseshoe fills the hollow around the lateral malleolus and prevents further swelling. (b) Completed bandage for acute inversion sprain of the ankle.

4. Repeat this manoeuvre, ensuring the bandage crosses at the level of the injured ligament each time. Also ensure that the heel is enclosed by the bandage so that fluid cannot accumulate.

5. Once the heel is enclosed and the ligament well supported, continue to enclose the lower leg, overlapping the bandage as you move proximally up the limb (Fig 3.2b).

Acute knee strapping – figure of eight wrap

When bandaging the injured knee, the temptation is simply to use a circular bandaging technique from distal to proximal over the knee joint. This form of bandaging may produce excessive compression of the region, including the patellofemoral joint, and commonly slips down the leg when the athlete moves.

A figure of 8 wrap produces effective compression, avoiding the patellar region, and remains in place very effectively.

Tape: 7.5 cm cohesive bandage or EAB

1. Start bandaging a reasonable distance below the knee, from the postero-lateral aspect of the limb and running anteriorly and medially (Fig 3.3a).

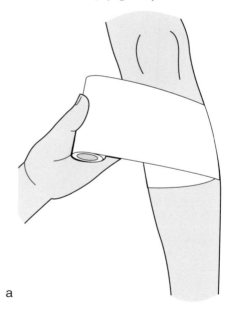

a

Fig 3.3 Figure of 8 wrap. (a) Starting position.

(Continued)

2. Complete a locking technique and then angle the
   bandage superiorly and medially over the medial joint
   line.
3. Run the bandage posteriorly and laterally behind the
   knee and then superiorly and medially over the anterior
   aspect of the femur (Fig 3.3b).

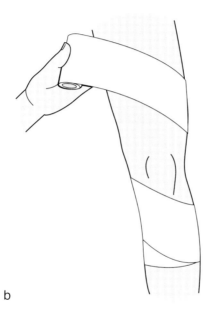

b

Fig 3.3—cont'd   (b) Bandage continues medially over the femur.

(Continued)

4. Continue to encircle the thigh and then bring the bandage inferiorly and medially down over the joint line staying above the patella as you do (Fig 3.3c). Run the bandage behind the knee, and then bring it anteriorly over the lateral joint line, angling it in a superior direction above the patellar and across the anterior thigh.

5. Continue around the thigh and down over the lateral joint line again, this time below the level of the patella and across the anterior shin (Fig 3.3d). This completes the full Figure of 8. Additional compression can be used as required.

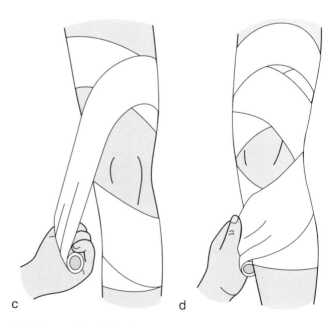

c   d

Fig 3.3—cont'd (c) Bandage runs inferiorly over the medial joint line, (d) Bandage runs inferiorly over the lateral joint line to complete the bandaging.

Intermittent compression therapy may be of value, using a variety of devices available on the market. However, it is not practical to use these forms of devices continually, and it is suggested that some form of alternative compression is used as well.

E levation

Elevating the injured body part above the level of the heart assists with venous return and limits excessive swelling. This notion is based on limited biological evidence, but is reasonably well supported by clinical research. As swelling can cause an increase in pressure within a body region, excessive swelling can be a source of mechanical pain and may contribute to the overall pain pattern in the patient's presentation.

Ideally, an injured limb should be elevated above the level of the heart as much as possible and as quickly as possible, for the first 72 hours post injury.

At all times, the clinician needs to monitor the effectiveness of the PRICE regime on the individual athlete and modify accordingly.

Range of motion

One essential element of improving function is the restoration of full range of motion to a joint or region. The goal, in terms of range, is best determined by comparing the injured region with the other, uninjured side and aiming for comparable pain-free motion. While major deficiencies in range are self evident, small, but functionally important losses in range are often overlooked during the rehabilitation programme and can severly limit progression.

There are numerous techniques that the clinician can use to improve range of motion. The effective technique will be the one that targets the structures causing the limitation of movement. Factors that cause a restriction in range include:

3

Treatment and Rehabilitation

- Swelling / oedema
- Muscle spasm / guarding
- Pain on movement
- Muscle / soft tissue tightness
- Joint stiffness – post immobilization or associated with degenerative changes

Techniques that target these factors are given below.

Swelling / oedema

- PRICE (see previous section)
- Use of electrophysical agents

Muscle spasm / guarding

- Contract / relax techniques (Fig 3.4)
- Hold / relax techniques – Muscle energy techniques

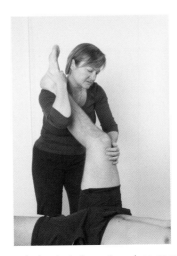

Fig 3.4   Contract / relax techniques to reduce muscle spasm.

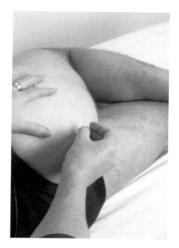

Fig 3.5 Dry needling to reduce trigger point activity and associated pain.

- Trigger point release
- Dry needling / intramuscular stimulation (IMS) (Fig 3.5)

Painful movement

- Cryotherapy
- Use of electrophysical agents
- Manual mobilization techniques
- Drug management and injection therapy

Muscle / soft tissue tightness

- Massage
- Stretching

Joint stiffness

- Manual mobilization techniques (see Figs 2.6 and 3.45)
- NAGS and SNAGs (see Fig 3.46)

NB: It is essential to ensure the accessory motion of a joint has also been restored and not just the physiological movement, e.g. Fig 3.6.

Any increase in range must be followed by appropriate exercises to both maintain the range gained, and also to develop muscle strength and control within this newly acquired range.

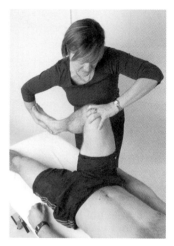

Fig 3.6 Accessory tibio/femoral rotation of the knee.

Movement diagrams

In order to utilize manual techniques most effectively, every clinician should be familiar with the concept of movement diagrams. "Drawing" a "mental movement diagram" for any joint or movement pattern is necessary to select the appropriate grade and rhythm of technique. A movement diagram forces clinicians to evaluate whether they are treating pain or stiffness, if the region is highly irritable, what the limiting factor to movement is and, from there, what technique will affect these factors in the most expedient fashion.

Further discussion of movement diagrams is beyond the scope of this book, but the reader is directed to Maitland G, Hengeveld E, Banks K and English K (2005) Vertebral Manipulation, 7th ed. Butterworth Heinemann, for more detailed information.

Muscle re-education / training

With the awareness of motor control problems in the manifestation of many musculoskeletal conditions, clinicians are increasingly focusing on re-education of movement patterns. Shirley Sahrmann has written an excellent text on this subject.

Sahrmann S (2001) Diagnosis and Treatment of Movement Impairment Syndromes. Mosby, St. Louis.

Correct technique and isolated activity are essential for performance, but once this foundation has been laid, the clinician must ensure that exercises are prescribed to increase muscular strength, endurance and power. Exactly how and to what extent these are addressed will depend on the athlete's sporting demands and the nature of their competitive season.

Strength

Strength refers to the amount of force a muscle is capable of producing in a single effort. It is determined by the size of the muscle fibres and the efficiency of the neural mechanisms activating the muscle.

3

Treatment and Rehabilitation

167

Resistance or weight training is the most common form of strength training. For strength gains to be achieved, the muscle must be worked slightly beyond its normal physiological capabilities. This causes subtle trauma to the muscle and results in an increase in the size of the muscle fibres. This is known as the overload principle. Strength training involves high loads and a low number of repetitions. As the muscle is pushed beyond its physiological capability, adequate rest periods are required between strength training sessions. Normally only 1−2 strength sessions are performed in a week.

The Oxford Scale of muscle strength

The Oxford Scale is used as a clinical tool for assessing and recording muscle strength. Muscle strength is rated on a scale from 0 to 5. The muscle is tested for its ability to produce movement of the associated joint in a specific direction and is determined by observation and palpation of the muscle belly and tendon.

0 – No discernible muscle action on observation or palpation of the muscle

1 – A muscle twitch is discernible, but does not result in any movement of the related joint or limb

2 – The muscle is capable of producing the appropriate full range joint movement, but only in a gravity-eliminated position

3 – The muscle is capable of producing full range movement of the joint against gravity

4 – The muscle is capable of producing the appropriate movement against some level of resistance but not to a level that the clinician judges to be normal.

5 – The muscle is capable of producing full range, non-compensatory movement against a normal level of resistance

What is "normal"?

This is a professional judgment based on what the clinician expects would be full muscle power for a particular individual. It is based on the health, age, activity level and weight of the individual. Clinicians working with teams and groups of athletes have an advantage in that they can establish baseline measurements of strength, endurance and power during screening. They can compare this data against measurements of muscle function post injury.

Kendall FP, Kendall EM, Provance PG, et al (2005) Muscles: Testing and Function, with Posture and Pain, 5th ed. Lippincott, Williams and Wilkins, Philadelphia.

Endurance

Endurance refers to the ability of a muscle to undergo repeated contractions against a set resistance for a period of time. It is an important component of fatigue and commonly features as a problem in overuse injuries.

A lighter weight with a higher number of repetitions is the basis for endurance training. Baseline testing for each individual athlete is essential to establish the appropriate starting weight and the number of repetitions.

Power

Power refers to a muscle's ability to produce high levels of force at high speeds. It is defined as the product of force and velocity. It is considered one of the most important variables in determining an athlete's performance in cases where athletes are involved in propulsive actions, such as sprinting or throwing.

In designing rehabilitation programmes, clinicians often fail to include exercises for power development. Neglecting this aspect of function will result in an athlete returning to training and playing ill-prepared for the demands of sporting competition.

Neuromuscular components are important in power development because of the speed dimension. This suggests that power training requires repetition of specific activities at speed. Plyometric drills such as vertical jumps, hopping and bounding, speed drills like shuttle sprints and explosive drills such as kicking are all good power activities for the lower limb. In the upper limb, boxing activities and

3

Treatment and Rehabilitation

throwing or swinging weighted objects (medicine balls / bar bells with the Smith machine) are good power drills.

In rehabilitating the injured athlete, communication between the therapist, coach and strength and conditioning trainer is essential to ensure the athlete undertakes a progressively demanding programme that includes all aspects of muscle function. A combination of rehabilitation and a return to training should occur as soon as possible. This is only achievable if effective communication exists between all members of the medical and coaching staff and a detailed rehabilitation and training programme is compiled which includes, every aspect of their expected activity.

Too often, little overlap exists between rehabilitation and training, and the athlete makes the transition from the physiotherapist's clinic to the gym environment with an excessive increase in physical demands, making the player vulnerable to overload and re-injury, or even the development of a new injury.

Proprioception

Deficits in proprioception (collection of the information exchanged between the sensory and motor systems regarding movement and the position of body parts) following injury are well documented as is evidence to show benefits of proprioceptive retraining on the prevention of reinjury. Injuries requiring surgery or immobilization tend to have greater proprioceptive deficits due to downtime and decreased use.

When an athlete sustains an injury to a body region, structures relating to the somatosensory system are also damaged. As a result, kinaesthetic acuity (the ability to detect motion) and joint position sense are diminished. This leads to reduced balance and co-ordination, prolonged muscular reaction times and decreased muscle strength, making the region less capable of reacting appropriately to imposed forces – commonly referred to as "instability". It is important to recognize that this is not osseo-ligamentous instability (though this may be present as well) but represents a functional instability.

As with all other aspects of rehabilitation, it is essential to have an objective measurement of proprioception to reassess progress. At the most basic level, this may be an indication of the time the athlete can maintain a stable position on one leg. A more functional and dynamic test is the Star Excursion Balance Test, described by Kinzey and Armstrong.

Kinzey SJ and Armstrong CW (1998) The Reliability of the Star-Excursion Test in Assessing Dynamic Balance. Journal of Orthopaedic and Sports Physical Therapy 27: 356–360.

Star Excursion Balance Test procedure

The test involves having the athlete stand and maintain their base of support on one leg while maximally reaching in different directions with the other leg along a testing grid in the form of a star as shown (Fig 3.7) The star shaped testing grid is formed by 8 lines, each 120 cm long, extending out

3

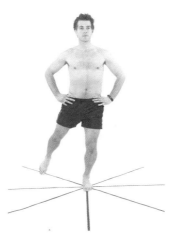

Fig 3.7 Star Excursion Balance Test set-up.

from a common point at a 45° angle. It can be created using standard sports tape laid on a smooth, firm surface.

Instruct the athlete to reach as far as possible along each of the eight lines, make a light touch on the line, and return the reaching leg back to the centre, while maintaining single-leg stance with the other leg in the centre of the star. Start with the anterior direction and work in a clockwise direction around the grid. Measure the distance along each line. Three trials in each direction are commonly utilized in testing, the scores averaged and added up for each limb.

Proprioceptive tests for the upper limb are lacking in the literature. The most commonly described test is an assessment of joint position sense in which the therapist places the uninjured limb into various positions and asks the athlete to mimic these with the injured limb (Fig 3.8). Objective tests of accuracy can be taken using a goniometer to measure differences in limb position.

In the upper limb, athletes that use the upper limb in an open chain pattern such as throwing and ball sports should perform proprioceptive training that focuses on this type of action. Similarly, if the athlete is involved in closed kinetic chain activities, such as gymnastics or kayaking, proprioceptive retraining must emphasize this component of movement.

Much of the research looking at proprioceptive retraining in the lower limb has involved subjects standing on wobble boards, and this has led to a lack of thought and imagination in proprioceptive training in the clinical environment. In the upper limb, very few retraining programmes are described.

Key elements of proprioceptive exercises include:

- Uncertainty
- Reaction speeds
- Distraction — focusing on tasks other than what is occurring at the region being exercised
- Precision in task performance
- Endurance
- Co-contraction and weight bearing

Something other than a wobble board! – ideas for proprioceptive training

- Mirror images – therapist places one limb in a position and asks the patient to replicate this with the injured limb (Fig 3.8a,b)
- Tracing tasks – following a pattern drawn on a wall / floor by the therapist using the injured limb
- Placement tasks – Star Excursion Balance Test – progress from stepping to hopping (Fig 3.9)
- Mini trampette – hopping on / hopping off
- BOSU ball – Step ups / step downs / lunges / small knee bends / push ups
- Hopscotch
- Ball work – throwing / catching / footwork
- Ladder work – increasing speed
- Dance mats

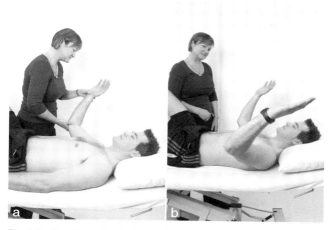

Fig 3.8 Proprioceptive tasks – mirror imaging: (a) start and (b) finish position.

3

Treatment and Rehabilitation

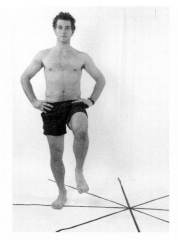

Fig 3.9 Proprioceptive tasks – hopping task for star excursion balance test.

Braces and supports

Rehabilitation

The use of braces and supports during the rehabilitation stage has very different objectives to their use for return to play and function.

During rehabilitation, braces are primarily designed to protect the damaged structures from re-injury and maintain the joint or structure in a position to optimize healing. They are often designed to limit joint range in a way that allows the range to be adjusted and increased as healing and rehabilitation progress. This is usually the case after surgery, such as ACL reconstruction or shoulder rotator cuff repair. Some surgeons may also recommend the use of a brace or support following a fracture or significant sprain to the wrist or hand. In most cases, the brace is used in the initial phases of rehabilitation when the cast has been removed and the joint is not well supported by muscular control.

While application of an abduction brace is common practice by surgeons following rotator cuff repair, use of braces and supports with injuries to the knee is very variable, dependent mainly on the practices and opinion of the surgeon or sports physician in non-operative cases such as Grade 2 MCL tears. There is a lack of research evidence that bracing for the knee has a significant effect on outcome following injury or surgery.

The other common form of bracing for rehabilitation is the use of "off loading braces" in degenerative conditions such as unicompartmental osteoarthritis of the knee. Dennis et al (2006) showed that the "OAdjuster" brace by DonJoy and the "Thruster" by Bledsoe are two of the most effective braces on the market in achieving separation between the medial condyles of the tibia and femur of the knee.

Dennis DA, Komistek RD, Nadaud MC et al (2006) Evaluation of off-loading braces for treatment of unicompartmental knee arthrosis. The Journal of Arthroplasty 21 (Suppl):2–8.

Function

Prophylactic braces are designed to prevent or minimize injury in the event of an accident. There is no evidence to support the use of braces or supports in this fashion.

The same style of brace is often used by athletes to support and protect previous injuries during training and competition. They are referred to as functional braces. The effects of these braces are:

- Mechanical – aiming to minimize potentially damaging movements in certain directions. The evidence for this is equivocal.
  - Abduction and external rotation control – anteriorly dislocating shoulder.
  - Valgus / varus and tibial rotation – post ACL reconstruction.

3

Treatment and Rehabilitation

- Proprioceptive – provide improved awareness of joint position. This has been demonstrated within the research laboratory; however studies have not been able to replicate the high levels of force and torsion that joints would be subjected to in most sporting activities. It is therefore difficult to determine the effect of braces on proprioception and support in "real life" situations.
- Psychological – give the athlete a sense of safety and reduced injury risk.

When considering the use of a functional brace for an athlete, emphasize to the athlete that braces and supports are never intended to be used in place of a comprehensive and well designed rehabilitation programme.

Some supports for joints and limbs primarily aid compression and retain heat. They offer little in the way of joint stability or motion control, but may act to "support" the area by improving proprioception or facilitating muscle function.

These supports are often made of neoprene and are often worn by recreational athletes who have purchased the products independently from sporting stores or online. They probably offer psychological support for the athlete as well. There is no evidence that their use is either beneficial or detrimental.

Returning to running

When starting to run again after a period of inactivity the athlete is often vulnerable to breakdown and re-injury. To start a running programme, it is generally accepted that an athlete must have sufficient quadriceps and calf strength of at least 80% of the unaffected limb. Consideration must also be given to the stage of tissue healing and repair.

Little evidence exists regarding the most effective way to implement and progress a running programme. Table 3.1 shows an example of a running programme used in clinical situations for individuals returning to running after an injury, post-operatively or following an overuse injury. For

Table 3.1 Return to running programme

Week	Exercise duration	Interval period	Interval breakdown
1	30 min	5 min	Walk 4 min Run 1 min
2	30 min	5 min	Walk 3 min Run 2 min
3	30 min	5 min	Walk 2 min Run 3 min
4	30 min	5 min	Walk 1 min Run 4 min
5	Run 30 min		

the most controlled environment this should be done on a treadmill before progressing to outside and more uneven surfaces.

This running programme can be easily altered in terms of the number of interval periods completed or the progression from one week to the next. In our clinic, we usually advise patients to perform this programme on alternate days, interspersing it with ongoing gym-based strength rehabilitation.

Signs that progression may be too fast:

- Development of an effusion
- Development of pain / soreness – need to differentiate from soreness associated with increasing levels of exercise
- Inability to progress with other exercises – strength

Once the athlete can complete a 30-minute running session comfortably, further progressions can be achieved by increasing the distance run in the same time (speed), increasing duration or increasing the uneven nature and type of terrain. These progressions will be goal driven depending on the activities the athlete is returning to.

From this point, the athlete enters the return to play stage of their rehabilitation programme which will be dealt with in the following section.

3

Treatment and Rehabilitation

Case studies

The following case studies are designed to show practical implementation of the principles discussed. The reader should also refer to the relevant section of the Assessment section that deals with the clinical findings for each condition.

In an ideal world, we would all work in a multidisciplinary team where specific elements of rehabilitation would each be dealt with by someone specialized in that field.

In the real world, this is rarely the case. To be more effective at those areas of rehabilitation where you feel less skilled, utilize every opportunity to observe, work and learn from other professions. A world-renowned sports physician told me he learnt most of his sport's medicine from working with physiotherapists, and I know that I and many other physiotherapists have developed new rehabilitation skills and programmes from working alongside strength and conditioning trainers, and improved our soft tissue work working with sports massage therapists.

Case study – Severe ankle sprain

A 19-year-old female netballer sustains an inversion injury of her left ankle while playing in a club competition. She is due to play an international match in 8 weeks' time and must report to the training camp a week prior to this. She is assessed court side and management is instigated at this point.

Presenting problems

Symptoms and signs

- Unable to weight bear on the leg – needs to be helped off the court
- Significant tenderness over the ligament and surrounding area
- Little swelling
- Limited range of motion
- Unable to assess ligamentous laxity due to pain level

Problems known to be associated with the pathology

- Loss of ligamentous integrity
- Loss of balance and proprioception
- Pain inhibition of peroneals with loss of strength and muscle bulk over time
- Loss of cardiovascular fitness

Phase 1: first 24 hours

Rehabilitation goals

1. Protect from further injury
2. Control swelling
3. Reduce pain
4. Facilitate tissue healing
5. Educate patient regarding condition, management plan and prognosis

Rehabilitation programme

PRICE – educate patient re PRICE regime

Brace / bandage to limit motion (see acute ankle bandaging Fig 3.2)

3

Treatment and Rehabilitation

Provide crutches for patient to mobilize NWB and educate regarding the use of crutches

Electrophysical agents, e.g. ultrasound, interferential

Discuss use of pain relief medication with medical officer

NB: NSAIDs are now used more judiciously for the relief of pain and swelling in soft tissue trauma due to their effects on the repair process.

Phase 2: 24–72 hours

With the provision of adequate pain relief and the instigation of the PRICE regime, ligamentous testing can be performed (see Fig 2.35). It is determined that the athlete has sustained a Grade 2 sprain of her anterior talo-fibular ligament (ATFL).

Rehabilitation goals

1. Continue to protect from further injury
2. Continue to control swelling
3. Reduce pain
4. Facilitate tissue healing
5. Maintain lower limb strength
6. Maintain upper body strength
7. Maintain CV fitness
8. Commence proprioceptive retraining

Rehabilitation programme

PRICE

Continue bandage and crutches

Pain medication as required – paracetamol

Electrophysical agents

Active knee flexion and extension in sitting – with ankle weights positioned around shin

Active knee flexion in prone and supine – with ankle weights

Bridging – single leg (Fig 3.10)

Hip abduction in side lying (Fig 3.11)

Hip extension in 4 pt (see Fig 3.26)

One leg standing – single leg squats for the unaffected limb

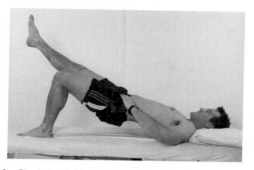

Fig 3.10 Single leg bridging.

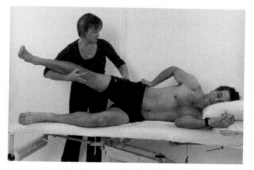

Fig 3.11 Hip abduction in side lying – ensure pelvis is in neutral position (avoid anterior rotation) and hip is extended.

Continue upper body conditioning programme

Standing balance exercises – uninjured limb (evidence of carry over to injured limb) See section on proprioception (p. 170).

Seated boxing / grinder

Phase 3: 72 hours – 1 week

Assess weight bearing ability. As rapidly as possible, the athlete should recommence weight bearing and walking with a normal gait pattern. The determining factor is the presence of pain during walking.

In this instance, the player was not comfortable mobilizing without the use of crutches, so was encouraged to walk normally while taking some weight through the crutches. She gradually reduced the amount of weight taken through the crutches until by the end of the 1st week post injury she was able to mobilize with a normal gait pattern, without the use of crutches.

Rehabilitation goals

Criteria for progression – no increase in pain or swelling.

1. Continue to control pain and swelling
2. Facilitate tissue healing
3. Restore normal gait pattern
4. Restore ROM to ankle
5. Limit strength loss around ankle
6. Continue to maintain upper and lower body strength
7. Continued re-education of proprioception
8. Maintain CV fitness

Rehabilitation programme

Continued bandaging and compression as necessary

Gait re-education / pool walking

Active ROM exercises for the ankle within the limits of pain

Manual mobilization techniques to improve dorsiflexion range (Fig 3.12)

Isometric strength exercises around the ankle

Proprioceptive work:

- alphabet writing with ankle (within the limits of pain)
- joint position sense exercises
- rhythmic stabilization exercises around the ankle
- swiss ball – single leg work (Fig 3.13)

Ongoing conditioning and CV work as above

Phase 4: 1–4 weeks

Rehabilitation goals

Criteria for progression – no pain or swelling

1. Full ROM
2. Increase ankle strength
3. Continue re-education of proprioception

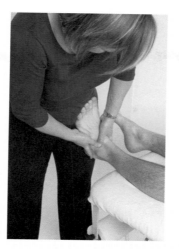

Fig 3.12 Manual mobilization techniques for the talocrural joint to improve dorsiflexion range of motion.

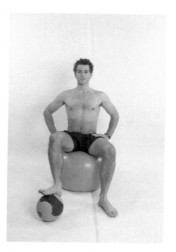

Fig 3.13 Sitting balance exercises to improve proprioception.

3

Treatment and Rehabilitation

4. Maintain CV fitness and strength
5. Maintain sports specific skills

Rehabilitation programme

Stop bandaging. Player may wear neoprene support for comfort

Dorsiflexion exercises in weight bearing (Fig 3.14)

Calf stretches

Double leg heel raises – progress to single leg raises as pain permits

Eversion exercises with theraband (resistance as pain permits) (Fig 3.15)

Plantar flexion exercises with theraband (resistance as pain permits)

Stepping sideways against theraband resistance applied to lateral tibia

Pool walking and running

Proprioceptive work

- commence balance training – single leg stance

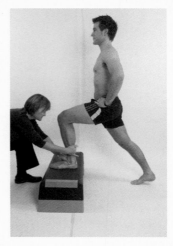

Fig 3.14 Exercise to improve ankle dorsiflexion range.

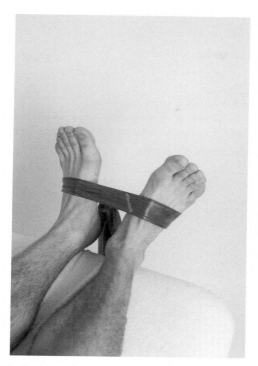

Fig 3.15 Ankle eversion strengthening exercises with theraband.

- wobble board work
- walking on uneven surfaces

(see generic proprioceptive training section at the beginning of this section)

CV work – cycling or swimming

Sport specific ball skills with coaching staff (stationary)

Phase 5: 4–7 weeks

Soft tissue healing occurs by week 6, but ongoing remodelling and reorganization of collagen fibres continues to occur for some time. Rehabilitation should aim for

3

Treatment and Rehabilitation

increasing function in an environment in which the healing structures are protected from further injury.

Rehabilitation goals

Criteria for progression – no pain or swelling

1. Full strength
2. Dynamic proprioceptive training
3. Return to running and restricted sport specific drills
4. Maintain CV fitness and strength

Rehabilitation programme

Commence run–walk programme – progress as pain permits, aiming for 30 minutes running by 6 weeks with increasing speed in weeks 7 and 8. This programme commenced on the treadmill and progressed in weeks 7 and 8 to uneven ground (see Table 3.1).

The player's strength and conditioning programme should become more dynamic and functional as the player tolerates increasing weight-bearing forces on the ankle:

- Strength work – lunges / squats
- Step ups
- Side step ups with weight (Fig 3.16a,b)
- Moving sideways up and down an incline - focus on lateral stability
- Progression to plyometric work – mini tramp / box jumps (Fig 3.17a,b)
- Proprioceptive retraining:
  - Ladder drills
  - Star excursion balance test (see Fig 3.7 and 3.9)
  - Hopping with control – on and off mini tramp
  - Hopscotch
  - Throwing / catching with netball – standing on injured leg, moving to catch the ball and landing on injured leg
- Commence speed and agility training:
  - Shuttle runs – change of direction
  - Weaving / figure of 8 runs (see Fig 4.6)
  - Ongoing sport specific skills – commence skills involving running and catching

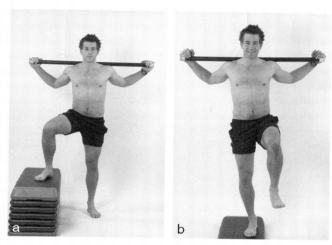

Fig 3.16 Side step ups with weight: (a) start and (b) finish position.

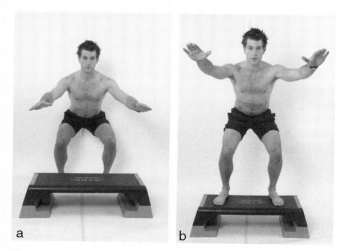

Fig 3.17 Plyometric training – box jumps showing (a) start and (b) finish position.

Phase 5: 7–8 weeks (training camp)

Rehabilitation goals

1. Full ROM, strength and endurance
2. Return to sport specific drills, training and match play

The athlete was monitored continually throughout the training camp for increases in pain and development of an effusion. She was able to complete all of the ball handling drills and was able to gradually increase the level of plyometric training she completed over the course of the week. The physiotherapist monitored her training and discussed with the coaching and conditioning staff any modifications. These included a reduction in the number of repetitions she undertook for each exercise and the distances she aimed for with plyometric activities. Over the course of the week, she increased these factors, using pain as a guide, until she was undertaking a full training programme by the end of the training camp.

In the course of the week, she underwent several Return to Play drills and was passed fit to compete in the competition. See section 4 for information on return to play.

Ankle braces for training / return to play

Netballers and basketballers who have sustained an injury to their ankle commonly employ either strapping or a brace when returning to play. A Cochrane review on the subject came to the conclusion that semi-rigid orthoses or air cast braces (see section on braces) can be effective at reducing the likelihood of athletes incurring a further sprain.

Handoll HHG, Rowe BH, Quinn KM, de Bie R (2001) Interventions for preventing ankle ligament injuries. Cochrane Database of Systematic Reviews Issue 3 Art. No: CD000018. Doi: 10.1002/14651858 .CD000018.

Clinical commentary

Research from animal studies now suggests that moderate ligamentous injuries (Grade 2) benefit from a short period of early immobilization to optimize the repair process. Following this, rehabilitation programmes need to emphasise proprioceptive retraining and plyometric work to prepare the athlete for a return to a sport involving rapid changes of direction.

Case study – Grade I tear of biceps femoris muscle

A 22-year-old elite male 400 m hurdler presents to a sports medicine clinic the day after experiencing a feeling of tearing / pulling while training. He is due to compete at the UK Athletic Championships in 2 weeks time. He had a similar problem 3 months previously from which he had recovered quickly with treatment. As instructed after the previous injury, he has iced the injury, sitting on an ice pack and actively flexing and extending his knee within the limits of discomfort.

He has full range of knee extension and is able to walk normally, with a feeling of tension / discomfort in the hamstring. He presents wearing compression shorts under his clothing.

Presenting problems

Symptoms and signs

- Tenderness over the musculo-tendinous junction of the long head of biceps femoris
- No evidence of bruising or swelling
- No restriction to knee range of motion, but some feeling of tightness and pain towards the end of single leg raise (SLR)
- Pain with resisted hamstring contraction
- Normal gait pattern

Problems known to be associated with the pathology

- Pain inhibition of hamstrings with loss of strength
- Loss of balance and proprioception
- Neural irritation
- Lumbo-pelvic dysfunction contributing to development of the pathology - often strength imbalance between hamstrings and gluteals or over activity in hamstring function
- Loss of cardiovascular fitness

Phase 1: 24–48 hours

As the athlete is an elite runner who has had previous problems, he undergoes an MRI scan of both his lumbar spine and his hamstring muscle. The MRI shows no pathology in the lumbar spine but evidence of a longitudinal tear of the biceps femoris in the region of the musculo-tendinous junction.

Discussions by the medical team (sports physician, physiotherapist, musculoskeletal radiologist, strength and conditioning trainer) concludes that he should be fit to compete in 2 weeks time. The rehabilitation programme focuses during this period on the injury signs and symptoms. Once he has competed in the Championships, his lumbo-pelvic control will be assessed and appropriate management instigated.

As the athlete is due to compete in 2 weeks time, strength gains in the hamstring muscle are not feasible. Exercise therapy aims to improve the neuromuscular control of the hamstring, progressing to strength and power gains after the Championships.

Rehabilitation goals

1. Protect from further injury
2. Control swelling / minimize bleeding
3. Reduce pain
4. Facilitate tissue healing
5. Restore neuromuscular control of the hamstrings
6. Maintain gluteal strength
7. Early re-education of proprioception
8. Maintain CV fitness

Rehabilitation programme

PRICE – active knee extension while sitting on an ice pack – 5 minutes

Electrophysical agents

Active knee flexion and extension in sitting with light theraband resistance

Active knee flexion in prone and supine – light theraband resistance / low reps (pain free)

Static, through range holds for 6 seconds

Commence eccentric programme – "wobbles" – low reps to avoid fatigue (Box 3.2)

Bridging
- Knees bent – heels on floor (Fig 3.18)
- Straight leg – heels on bed

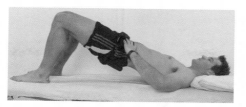

Fig 3.18 Double leg bridging.

Box 3.2 Eccentric hamstring training

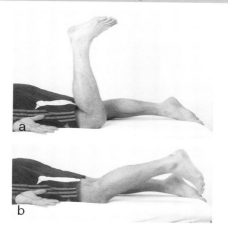

Fig 3.19 Eccentric hamstring training – Flicks showing (a) start and (b) finish position.

- **Flicks (Fig 3.19a,b)**

  The athlete lies prone with their knee bent to 90°

  They rapidly extend their lower leg towards the floor and then flex the lower limb quickly as the foot contacts the floor, as though trying to "flick" their toe against the floor

3

Treatment and Rehabilitation

- **Catches**

  Lying prone with the knee bent to 90°

  The athlete allows the lower limb to fall towards the floor, "catching" it by activating the hamstring muscles just before the toes hit the floor. The knee is then bent back to 90° and the exercises repeated

- **Wobbles**

  Lying prone with the knee bent to 90°

  The athlete flexes the lower limb from 90 to 100° flexion and then extends the knee to 80°. They continue to "wobble" the lower limb in this fashion until they feel their hamstring fatiguing

  These exercises are all performed until the hamstring fatigues

  Progression is achieved by

  - performing the exercises in standing
  - increasing the length at which the hamstring is activating by bending forwards at the hip over a table or bench (Fig 3.20a,b)

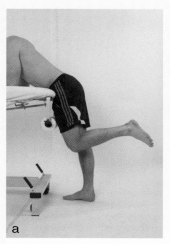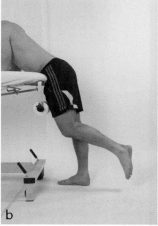

Fig 3.20 Eccentric hamstring training – progression showing (a) start and (b) finish position.

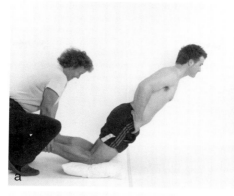

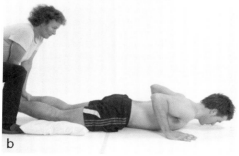

3

Fig 3.21 Nordic drills showing (a) start and (b) mid position.

- **Nordic drills**

  This exercise starts with the athlete in a kneeling position with their torso upright and the feet and ankles held rigidly by the therapist or coach

  The athlete begins the exercise by slowly lowering their torso towards the ground, using their hamstring muscles to control the descent. They maintain the eccentric contraction of the muscle for as long as possible before lowering themselves towards the floor with their hands

  From the floor, they push themselves back into a kneeling position, using their hamstrings concentrically to return to the starting position (Fig 3.21a,b)

Single leg balance exercises – STAR excursion balance exercise (see Fig 3.7)

Neural mobilization exercises – slump / SLR as tolerated (see Figs 2.22 and 2.40)

Swimming with a float between the legs

Gentle cycling (pain free)

Phase 2: 48–72 hours

Rehabilitation goals

Criteria for progression – no discomfort walking.

1. Facilitate tissue healing
2. Maintain ROM and neural mobility
3. Restore neuromuscular control of the hamstrings
4. Maintain strength in gluteals / quadriceps / core
5. Ongoing re-education of proprioception
6. Maintain CV fitness

Rehabilitation programme

Ongoing active ROM exercises / neural mobilization exercises – progress to controlled active ROM in standing – leg swings using alternating lead leg

Exercise therapy
- increase repetitions
- increase weight

Leg press machine

Progress bridging by increasing to:
- Single leg work (see Fig 3.10)
  - Swiss ball
  - Increasing holding time
  - Increasing number of repetitions

Continue proprioceptive work (see generic section on proprioception)

Maintain CV fitness
- Pool running
- Incline walking
- Cycling – increase resistance as pain permits

Phase 3: 72 hours–1 week

Rehabilitation goals

Criteria for progression – able to perform resisted hamstring contraction pain free.

1. Full ROM
2. Ongoing hamstring re-education
3. Continue re-education of proprioception
4. Return to light jogging
5. Maintain CV fitness

Rehabilitation programme

Progress hamstring work to include eccentric hamstring exercises

Single knee bends

Squats

Bridging – single leg $\pm$ Swiss ball (see Fig 3.10)

Plyometric work – hopping / bounding – gradually increase height and distance (see Fig 4.9)

Proprioceptive work:

- single leg standing
- tug of war (Fig 3.22), slapping (Fig 3.23) and joint position sense (Fig 3.24a,b)

Maintain CV fitness as listed above

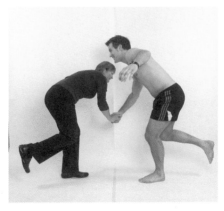

Fig 3.22   Proprioceptive training tug of war.

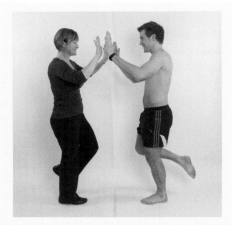

Fig 3.23 Proprioceptive training – single leg balance with destabilizing forces, slapping.

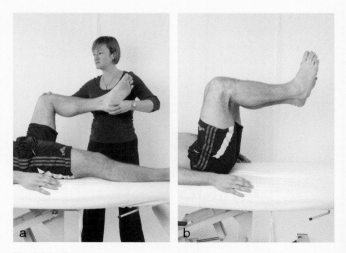

Fig 3.24 Proprioceptive training – joint position sense showing (a) start and (b) mirroring.

Jogging

Once the athlete is able to maintain full range of motion, walk pain free and perform a pain free resisted hamstring contraction against light resistance, they should commence gentle jogging.

Start at a gentle pace (50% of normal jogging pace) and gradually increase both distance and speed (do not increase both in the same session).

Once the athlete can jog for 1 km at approximately 70% of their normal pace, they should commence an acceleration / deceleration programme to work on the motor control of the hamstring muscle group.

There are many variations on the programme listed in Box 3.3. They all work towards the goal of restoring or improving the muscle's ability to adapt to changes in speed.

Phase 4: 1–2 weeks

Rehabilitation goals

1. Return to sport-specific drills
2. Return to training

The athlete is ready to resume training once the following criteria have been satisfied:

a. Completed running programme
b. Able to run forwards and backwards
c. Able to run up and downhill
d. Able to slow down and stop suddenly
e. Able to jump and hop
f. Able to complete all exercises with 100% confidence

Rehabilitation programme

Strength work – lunges (Fig 3.25) / squats

Step ups

Progression of plyometric work – mini tramp / box jumps (see Fig 3.17a,b)

3

Treatment and Rehabilitation

Box 3.3   Acceleration / deceleration programme

4 cones are placed so that a distance of 100m is broken into the following zones:

40m   20m   40m

Start the athlete running at 70% of maximum pace:

40 m - Accelerate up to 70% maximum pace

20 m - Maintain 70% pace

40 m - Decelerate to stop

- The athlete performs the task and then walks back to the starting cone
- The task is repeated twice
- If the athlete remains pain free, the outer cones are brought in 5 m, thus reducing the distance over which the athlete accelerates and decelerates, and the task is repeated twice more
- This process continues with a 5 min rest period between every 3 sets, until the athlete becomes "aware" of his / her hamstring
- At this time, the programme is ceased for the day. The athlete can continue the programme as long as they remain pain free and they do not have a sense of fatigue in their hamstring
- The following day, start the process from the beginning. The athlete should be capable of achieving more sets each day
- Once the acceleration / deceleration distance has been reduced to 5 m, the programme starts from the beginning at 90% of maximum pace and then again at 100%
- This programme should be undertaken on a 2 days on / 1 day off basis. (There are also various recommendations for this in existence. All athletes should be monitored for signs of fatigue)

Post competition rehabilitation

Prior to competition, the emphasis of the rehabilitation programme was on hamstring repair and neuromuscular control. Post competition, it is essential to address any overall motor control problems which may contribute to recurrent strains.

These athletes commonly present with lumbo-pelvic / hip dysfunction. Poor gluteal activation is coupled with overactivity of the hamstring and erector spinae, leading to overload of the low lumbar spine and excessive hamstring activation.

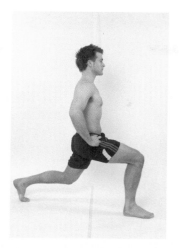

Fig 3.25 Lunges.

Rehabilitation goals

1. Motor control retraining
   - hamstrings / gluteals
   - gluteals / erector spinae (Fig 3.26)
   - hip dissociation with stable pelvis (Fig 3.26a)
   - hip extension (Fig 3.26)
   - hip extension with knee flexion (Fig 3.26c)

Rehabilitation programme

Release / downtraining work for hamstrings and erector spinae:

- Soft tissue work
- Active release techniques
- Muscle energy techniques
- Stretches (Fig 3.27)

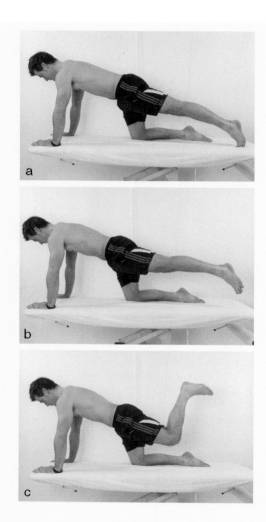

Fig 3.26 Motor control retraining – Gluteals vs. erector spinae

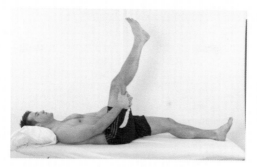

Fig 3.27 Hamstring stretches.

Specific dissociation exercises for gluteals:

- Hip extension in 4pt kneeling (see Fig 3.26)
- Squats / sit to stand (Fig 3.28)
- Roll downs
- Step ups
- Lunges (see Fig 3.25)

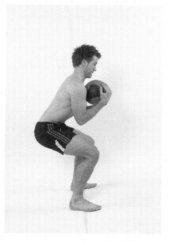

Fig 3.28 Squatting.

3

Treatment and Rehabilitation

Clinical commentary

Previous rehabilitation programmes for hamstring tears often focused on strengthening the hamstring, as the tear was considered an indication of muscle weakness.

However, recent work suggests two other factors may be at play:

- A neural component associated with dysfunction / "irritation" of the low lumbar spine leading to altered firing of the hamstring muscle. Some patients have a very positive SLR, which may also be associated with neural irritation at the level of the tear due to bleeding. Many athletes with recurrent hamstring problems have responded well to the use of a spinal epidural as part of their rehabilitation programme
- Altered motor control patterns for firing of the erector spinae, gluteals and hamstrings that may actually result in excessive hamstring activity (too STRONG rather than too weak).

 Sahrmann (2001) Diagnosis and Treatment of Movement Impairment Syndromes. St. Louis, Mosby.

In most patients with hamstring strains, it is a bit of "chicken and egg" situation as you often see evidence of all of these dysfunctions. Effective treatment requires all areas to be addressed.

Case study – Grade 2 strain of the medial collateral ligament

A 29-year-old female presents to a Sports Medicine clinic within 6 hours of experiencing a significant fall while skiing on-piste after a recent snowfall of approximately 1 m. She is diagnosed with a Grade 2 strain of her MCL. She is keen to return to amateur running, having signed up for a 10 km "fun run" in 14 weeks time.

Presenting problems

Symptoms and signs

- Significant tenderness over the ligament and surrounding area
- Mild swelling (effusion)

- Limited range of motion
- Ligamentous laxity

Problems known to be associated with the pathology

- Loss of ligamentous integrity
- Loss of balance and proprioception
- Pain inhibition of quadriceps with loss of strength and muscle bulk over time
- Loss of cardiovascular fitness

Phase 1: 0–2 weeks

Rehabilitation goals

1. Protect from further injury
2. Control swelling
3. Reduce pain
4. Facilitate tissue healing
5. Restore flexion range to 90°
6. Allow +20 knee extension, i.e. do not work into the last 20 degrees of full extension
7. 3/5 quadriceps strength (see muscle re-education section)
8. 4/5 hamstring strength
9. Maintain gluteal strength
10. Maintain CV fitness

Rehabilitation programme

PRICE

Hinged brace – locked 20–90 degrees

Electrophysical agents

Manual therapy

- physiological flexion mobilizations
- patellofemoral mobilizations in both neutral and knee flexion

Isometric quadriceps and SLR within the brace – 5–10 second holds is suggested as optimal for isometric contractions. The clinician needs to determine the number of repetitions based on observation of the athlete's performance of the exercise. When the athlete's performance becomes less than optimal, the muscle is fatiguing. This is the number of repetitions the athlete should perform.

Active knee flexion and extension in sitting

Active knee flexion in prone and supine – light theraband resistance

Bridging (see Figs 3.10 and 3.18)

Hip abduction in side lying (Fig 3.29)

Hip extension with theraband (tied proximally to the knee)

Seated boxing / grinder

Phase 2: 2–4 weeks

Rehabilitation goals

Criteria for progression – no swelling

1. No swelling
2. Facilitate tissue healing
3. Full flexion ROM
4. Allow +10 knee extension
5. 4/5 quadriceps strength
6. 4+/5 hamstring strength
7. Early re-education of proprioception
8. Maintain CV fitness

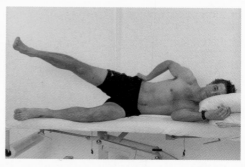

Fig 3.29 Hip abduction in side lying for gluteus medius strength.

Rehabilitation programme

Continued bracing and compression – alter brace settings
+10° extension – full flexion ROM

Active ROM exercises

Exercise therapy – low repetitions / high sets – minimize
irritation and swelling

Resisted hamstrings – theraband / leg weights

Leg press machine

Bridging

Swiss ball roll-outs

Active hip adduction against gravity

Commence cycling – gradual increase in resistance as pain
allows. Seat lowered to ensure +10° knee extension
maintained

Phase 3: 4–6 weeks

Rehabilitation goals

Criteria for progression – no swelling and full ROM

1. Full ROM
2. 4+/5 quadriceps strength
3. 5/5 hamstring strength
4. 5/5 adductor strength
5. Continue re-education of proprioception
6. Return to light jogging
7. Maintain CV fitness

Rehabilitation programme

Gait re-education

Full SLR – no active lag

Weight shift / single leg stance – ensure quadriceps activity in
inner range - add medial and lateral theraband resistance to
thigh as functional control permits

Single knee bends

Squats

Bridging – single leg ± swiss ball

Adduction exercises with theraband (NB: keep resistance proximal)

Jogging – see section "Return to running"

Cycling / cross trainer / stair master for CV work

Phase 4: 6–10 weeks

Rehabilitation goals

Criteria for progression – 4+quadriceps strength

1. Full ROM
2. Full strength
3. Power development
4. Full squat
5. Dynamic proprioceptive training
6. Return to running and restricted sport-specific drills

Rehabilitation programme

Strength work – lunges (see Fig 3.25) / squats (see Fig 3.28) / rotational lunges

Step ups

Side step ups with weight (see Fig 3.16a,b)

Progression to plyometric work – mini tramp / box jumps (see Fig 3.17a,b)

Change of direction training – shuttle runs / grid work / ladder work

Phase 5: 10+ weeks

Rehabilitation goals

Criteria for progression – full quadriceps strength

1. Good muscle endurance
2. Return to sport-specific activities

Rehabilitation programme

By this stage, the athlete should be commencing more sport-specific activities. In this case, running is the predominant activity. Common errors in the training programme of runners include the lack of a strength programme, cross training and a rest day. At this stage in the patient's rehabilitation, she was referred to a strength and conditioning trainer for discussion of an appropriate programme to cover the 4 weeks leading up to the race, and then the setting of new goals and a programme for future events.

Clinical commentary

It can sometimes be difficult when dealing with the recreational athlete to ensure they undertake a comprehensive rehabilitation programme that equips them for a safe return to activity. Once a patient is free from pain, keeping them focused is essential, and for this it is vital that the patient understands the goals and time frames of their rehabilitation programme.

Case study – medial tibial stress syndrome

A 34-year-old male banker decides to run the London Marathon, scheduled to take place this year on April 25th. He has a place running for charity and is very keen to complete the event. He started training on January 1st (as part of his New Year's resolutions) having only previously run as part of a regular gym programme that involved using the CV equipment and some upper body weights. His marathon training programme has consisted of running 5 days a week, steadily increasing the distance.

For the past two weeks, he has been experiencing pain in the medial aspects of his shins bilaterally, though his right shin is significantly worse than his left. These symptoms are present when he starts running, settle a little after he has run a couple of kilometres, but then get worse again at about 5 km. At present he is running 15 km, 5 days a week. He feels his symptoms are worsening and is concerned that he is not going to be able to compete in 4 weeks time.

3

Treatment and Rehabilitation

Presenting problems

Symptoms and signs

- Symptoms are present bilaterally. Significant, but non-specific tenderness along the medial border of both tibia
- Shin pain present running on treadmill but able to walk pain free
- No night pain
- Bilateral calf tightness with restricted ankle dorsiflexion
- Poor control of hip extension and external rotation in single leg stance
- Tight ITB
- Poorly developed quadriceps
- Poor balance in single leg stance

Problems known to be associated with the pathology

- Loss of cardiovascular fitness associated with inability to train / run
- Overpronation – increased stress on the tibialis posterior and traction of the tibial periosteum
- Rigid supinated foot – the lack of foot mobility results in poor force attenuation and the transmission of forces further up the lower limb.
- Periosteal inflammation

NB: When running on the treadmill, it appeared that this patient has a tendency to overpronate at the midtarsal joint. However, when the foot structure is examined, it is apparent that this was not the cause of the overpronation.

Examination of single leg stance illustrated poor control of the hip joint. Facilitation of the gluteus medius and maximus to improve hip extension / abduction and external rotation control reduced the overpronation evident at the foot.

When addressing biomechanical factors, it is essential to correlate the physical findings to the patient's symptoms to ensure treatment is specific and targeted, rather than a recipe / one size fits all approach (see Table 2.1 for more detail)

Phase 1: week 1

Rehabilitation goals

1. Protect from further injury
2. Education regarding condition and criteria for participation in the London Marathon
3. Maintain CV fitness
4. Facilitate tissue healing
5. Improve quadriceps strength
6. Improve gluteal strength
7. Release ITB / calves

Rehabilitation programme

Review of training programme:
- load modification / rest days
- CV work alternated with strength training – 1 rest day
- add strength work
- add flexibility work – stretching programme
  - dynamic warm up
- cross training (see CV work below)
- training surfaces

Check footwear:
- age and condition of running shoes
- appropriateness for foot type

Educate the patient regarding:
- this is an "overuse injury" and what that means
- this is not a "no pain – no gain scenario"
- the consequences of continuing with his current training regime
- the problems with his current training regime
- "realistic goal setting" – decision made in the week before the event, in response to treatment

Non impact CV work (must not provoke symptoms) – cross trainer / bike / boxing / rower / pool running with aqua jogger

Ice massage

Electrophysical agents

Soft tissue release work – calf and ITB

Quadriceps strength:

- squats (see Fig 3.28)
- lunges (see Fig 3.25)
- step ups
- one leg standing – small knee bends

Gluteal strength:

- hip extension in 4pt (see Fig 3.26a)
- hip abduction in side lying (see Fig 3.29)
- side step ups (see Fig 3.16)

Phase 2: weeks 2 and 3

Rehabilitation goals

Criteria for progression – no increase in pain level / able to undertake impact work pain free – must reassess running tolerance

1. Continue to maintain CV fitness
2. Continue to facilitate tissue healing
3. Continue strength work
4. Continue flexibility programme
5. Commence modified impact work

Rehabilitation programme

Increase duration of CV work – non-impact

Run / walk programme – if tolerated

Fartlek / interval training

Start power work for gluteals and quadriceps – plyometric:

- Mini tramp – jump squats
- Split squats
- Hopping

Plyometric exercise in the swimming pool:

- Running
- Hopping
- Jumping

- Bounding
- Split squats

Phase 3: week 4

Rehabilitation goals

Criteria for progression – preparation for marathon event

1. Continue to maintain CV fitness
2. Continue to facilitate tissue healing
3. Continue strength work
4. Continue flexibility programme
5. Decision regarding participation in London Marathon

Rehabilitation programme

CV work – swim

Use of ice massage

Gentle strength session × 2

Soft tissue release work

Marathon preparation

- Run / walk regime for event
- Nutrition – pre-event, during and post
- Hydration
- Warm up / Cool down
- Recovery – post event / next day

Clinical commentary

While the patient's aim is to complete the marathon at the end of week 4, it is unlikely that his symptoms will have resolved fully. New rehabilitation goals must be set, based on the patient's remaining signs and symptoms and his ongoing exercise plans.

If he simply wants to return to his regular gym programme, he should continue on the run / walk programme in association with the strength and stretching programme he has been undertaking. It is worth suggesting he speaks to the trainers at the gym regarding specific hip

3

Treatment and Rehabilitation

extensor / abductor exercises he can undertake to improve his lower limb biomechanics.

If he is keen to increase his level of competitive running, targeted events should be identified and a training programme instigated that includes a structured mileage increase, adequate rest days, cross training and an appropriate strength and conditioning programme. Warn him that many of the training programmes found on the internet or in magazines are designed for serious recreational runners, and that novice runners probably require about 6 months' preparation and training to run a marathon safely and effectively.

Interval training

Interval training is an important component of any athlete's rehabilitation or training programme. All athletes should cross train to minimize the risk of injury and overtraining. Interval work can form a very effective part of a cross training programme.

In the rehabilitation stage, a run / walk programme allows the injured athlete to challenge their injury in a low risk state, gradually increasing the duration and intensity of the activity over time.

For an athlete in training, interval work allows them to regulate workload, heart rate intensity and rates of recovery. It improves lactic tolerance and develops more efficient oxygen consumption by challenging both the aerobic and anaerobic systems.

Interval training can also help prevent the repetitive overuse injuries often associated with endurance activities, and allow an increase in training intensity with a smaller risk of overtraining.

What is Fartlek training?

Many runners are now incorporating this form of training into their schedules. Fartlek is a form of interval training that is not restricted by time or distance.

Fartlek sessions are more unstructured and are based on how the body feels and responds. Beginner runners often enjoy Fartlek work because it is not as demanding as other rigid interval sessions.

Fartlek work can be easily incorporated into a normal run around the park or local area. Runners simply increase their pace for a period or distance that feels comfortable, varying both speed and distance throughout the session. Objects such as streetlights, or distances such as the end of the road can be used to mark the faster segments.

Once a faster segment has been completed, the runner slows to a normal running pace until their breathing returns to a normal level.

Case study – recurrent shoulder dislocation

A 32-year-old female presents to physiotherapy for conservative management of a shoulder that has dislocated repeatedly on at least 6 occasions. On this occasion she has dislocated the shoulder diving into a swimming pool. She is an enthusiastic swimmer, currently training for an Olympic distance triathlon. On diving into the swimming pool, she felt the shoulder "pop out", but managed to relocate the shoulder herself. It was extremely sore, so she took some paracetamol and ibuprofen (an over-the-counter non steroidal anti-inflammatory drug).

Through her GP, she made an appointment to see an orthopaedic consultant the day after the injury. She discussed with the consultant the pros and cons of surgery versus conservative management. She had previously been treated conservatively and decides to trial conservative management again, as she is reluctant to have surgery.

She attends her first physiotherapy appointment a week after the incident.

3

Treatment and Rehabilitation

Presenting problems

Symptoms and signs

- Mild tenderness over the shoulder capsule and surrounding area
- Limited range of motion – flexion / abduction / external rotation / hand behind back – protective muscle spasm
- Ligamentous laxity – inferior and middle glenohumeral ligament
- Weak shoulder musculature

Problems known to be associated with the pathology

- Loss of proprioception around the shoulder
- Pain inhibition of rotator cuff and scapula function
- Loss of CV fitness

Phase 1: 0–2 weeks

Rehabilitation goals

1. Educate the swimmer regarding:
   - the aims and realistic expectations from conservative management
   - the importance of proprioceptive training versus strength training
2. Protect from further injury
3. Increase shoulder range of motion
4. Improve proprioception around the shoulder girdle
5. Improve motor control of the rotator cuff / glenohumeral joint
6. Improve motor control of the scapular musculature
7. Maintain CV fitness

Education – with this patient, it is extremely important to ensure she has realistic expectations of conservative management. She has previously worked through a conservative management programme, but her shoulder has continued to dislocate and she needs to be made aware that this may occur again, despite diligent work on a rehab programme. This information should have been provided to her by the orthopaedic consultant; however it requires reinforcing by the physiotherapist, so that the patient is not angry and frustrated if conservative management fails.

The patient also needs to be educated regarding the importance of proprioceptive retraining around the shoulder girdle to enhance movement control. Specific strength training is important, but needs to be built on an underlying basis of control to enhance joint stability.

Rehabilitation programme

Manual therapy

- physiological flexion mobilizations with AP accessory glide on the head of the humerus
- glenohumeral abduction with longitudinal accessory glide (see Fig 2.6)

Soft tissue techniques – pectorals / biceps / levator scapulae to reduce muscle overactivity

Contract/relax techniques to increase external rotation in neutral

Isolated rotational control of the glenohumeral joint (Fig 3.30)

Range of motion exercises:

- pendular techniques
- assisted active shoulder flexion

Isometric rotator cuff exercises

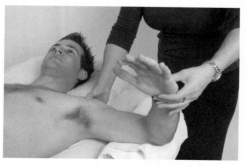

Fig 3.30   Exercise for isolating glenohumeral rotational control.

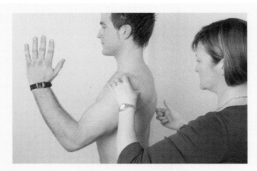

Fig 3.31 Dissociation exercises – isolating glenohumeral movement while maintaining a stable scapular position – flexion.

Specific scapular setting exercises including a focus on upward scapular rotation with serratus anterior activation

Dissociation exercises – flexion / abduction / external rotation (Fig 3.31)

Rhythmic stabilization work for the shoulder – proprioception (Fig 3.32)

Commence weight bearing exercise:
- against the wall
- double arm push ups
- single arm weight bearing

CV fitness:
- running / cycling
- Swimming – backstroke kicking with board at chest level

Phase 2: 2–4 weeks

Rehabilitation goals

1. Facilitate tissue healing
2. Full shoulder ROM
3. 4/5 rotator cuff strength
4. 4+/5 scapular strength
5. Ongoing re-education of proprioception
6. Maintain CV fitness

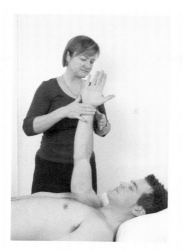

Fig 3.32 Proprioceptive training - rhythmic stabilization work for the shoulder.

Rehabilitation programme

Active ROM exercises

Exercise therapy – low repetitions / high sets – minimize irritation and swelling (Fig 3.33)

Proprioception – joint position "mirroring" (see Fig 3.8a,b)

Progress to weight bearing in a 4 pt kneeling position – rhythmic stabilization

CV work:

- can progress to exercise involving shoulders – cross trainer / rower
- Swimming – prone kicking with board in front (shoulder ROM permitting)

Phase 3: 4–6 weeks

Rehabilitation goals

Criteria for progression – full ROM

1. Full ROM
2. 4+/5 Rotator cuff strength

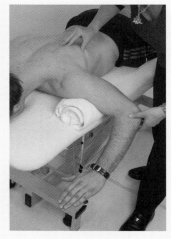

Fig 3.33 Anti gravity motor retraining for the rotator cuff.

3. 5/5 Scapular strength
4. Continue re-education of proprioception
5. Maintain CV fitness

Rehabilitation programme

Strength work – pool based programme – use of paddles / floats

Free weight and theraband work – rotational exercises / diagonal exercises (Figs 3.34 and 3.35)

Shoulder press – with hand weights

Lateral raises – with hand weights

Weight bearing exercise – push ups / superman

Balance on wobble board / small medicine ball (Fig 3.36)

CV work – add other water based components – aqua jogging

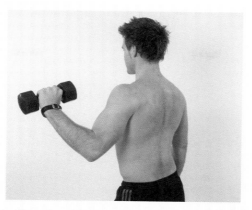

Fig 3.34 Strength training for the shoulder complex – compound exercises involving rotational movements.

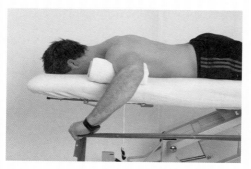

Fig 3.35 External rotation of the shoulder in abduction.

3

Treatment and Rehabilitation

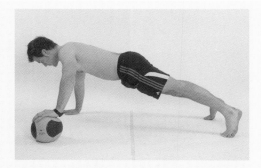

Fig 3.36 Proprioceptive training – push ups with medicine ball.

Phase 4: 6–8 weeks

Rehabilitation goals

Criteria for progression – 4+ strength

1. Full strength
2. Power development
3. Dynamic proprioceptive training

Rehabilitation programme

Plank holds (Fig 3.37)

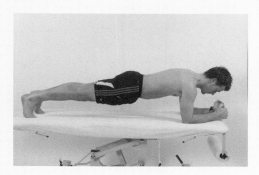

Fig 3.37 Plank hold.

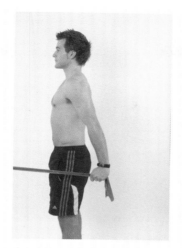

Fig 3.38 Strength training – posterior deltoid.

Strength work

- seated row
- biceps curl
- triceps push down
- lateral flys
- extension pulls (Fig 3.38)

Theraband exercises – prone rotation

Medicine ball – throwing / catching / swinging (Fig 3.44)

Smith machine – throwing / catching the bar

Phase 5: 8+ weeks

Rehabilitation goals

Criteria for progression – normal scapulohumeral rhythm

1. Full ROM, strength and endurance
2. Return to swimming training – need to build endurance and fatigue resistance
3. Continue proprioceptive retraining under fatigued conditions

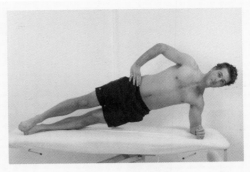

Fig 3.39 Compound exercises for the shoulder complex – rotating plank.

Rehabilitation programme

Rotating plank (Fig 3.39)

Balance work with gym ball / fitter

Endurance work for scapular and rotator cuff musculature

Boxing – glove and pad work – an excellent form of endurance exercise for the rotator cuff

Post exercise – rhythmic stabilizations / joint position sense

Clinical commentary

This patient needs to be aware that an ongoing strength and conditioning programme will be necessary to protect and support her shoulder, as well as the likelihood of re-injury. It is important for her to recognize that simply swimming will not keep her shoulder strong, and may potentially increase the chances of re-injury as a result of altered motor control. A comprehensive programme will ensure good neuromuscular function of the shoulder region.

Case study – shoulder impingement

A 24-year-old professional tennis player presents with a 6-week history of right shoulder pain that has resulted in withdrawal from the most recent tournament. She is scheduled to play in a tournament next week and then has a 2-week break before her next one.

Presenting problems:

Symptoms and signs

- Intermittent catching pain in the right shoulder associated with overhead activities with a constant low level dull ache
- Slight discomfort sleeping on right side
- Reproduction of symptoms with arm elevation – flexion and abduction
- Restricted hand behind back motion
- Protracted and downwardly rotated scapulae bilaterally (R) > (L)
- Anteriorly displaced head of humerus

Problems known to be associated with the pathology

- Inflammation of and microtrauma to cuff tendons
- Weakness and pain inhibition of the rotator cuff
- Loss of CV fitness

Phase 1: 0–1 week

A discussion must be had involving the player, her coach and her agent regarding the nature of her condition and the importance of playing in either or both of the upcoming tournaments.

All individuals need to be aware that ongoing tennis will aggravate and may worsen the condition. Treating the condition effectively will require rest from the aggravating elements of the game (overhead strokes / serving).

If the first tournament is essential, referral to a sports physician or extended scope physiotherapist for consideration of an injection of local anaesthetic / corticosteroid should be undertaken. It needs to be emphasized by all medical staff that this injection will not cure the problem, but would allow the player to play and perform her exercise programme in an effective pain-free fashion.

Non steroidal anti-inflammatory medication (Diclofenac / Brufen) may also be considered by the sports physician.

3

Treatment and Rehabilitation

It may be appropriate for the player to withdraw from the first tournament to focus on her rehabilitation, with the aim of playing fully fit in the second tournament.

In this instance, the player elected to play in the first tournament and then review her progress before the second. She had an injection by a sports physician and then had intensive daily physiotherapy treatment. Because of time limitations before playing, treatment focused on releasing tight and overactive structures to improve biomechanics.

Rehabilitation goals

1. Educate the patient and her coach regarding the condition, management and prognosis
2. Reduce pain
3. Release tight / overactive structures
4. Improve proprioceptive awareness of scapulothoracic posture and movement
5. Improve proprioceptive awareness of glenohumeral position and movement control
6. Commence biomechanical correction
7. Check cervical and thoracic spine
8. Maintain CV fitness

Rehabilitation programme

Injection plus NSAIDs

Education regarding condition

Soft tissue work:
- Posterior capsule (Fig 3.40)
- Pectoralis minor / major
- Subscapularis
- Biceps
- Levator scapulae

Stretches – internal glenohumeral rotation at 90 degrees

Motor control retraining – scapular positioning – upward rotation

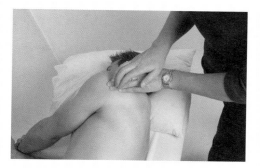

Fig 3.40 Soft tissue work to release the posterior components of the shoulder complex – muscle and capsule.

Glenohumeral rotation control in supine and standing (see Fig 3.30)

Cervical and thoracic range of motion exercises.

Manual mobilisation of cervical and thoracic spine to reduce any regions of hypomobility

Running programme / interval work

Footwork training – hurdles / ladder work

Phase 2: tournament 1–2 weeks

Throughout the tournament, the player continued to receive daily soft tissue work and undertook the exercise programme focusing on re-education of her motor control.

Phase 3: weeks 2–4

Rehabilitation goals

Criteria for progression – reduced pain level.

1. Facilitate tissue healing
2. Continue biomechanical correction – scapula and rotator cuff
3. Continue to release tight / overactive structures
4. Continue proprioceptive re-education
5. Maintain CV fitness
6. Review of technique with coach and player

3

Treatment and Rehabilitation

Rehabilitation programme

Use of taping to assist motor retraining – upward scapular rotation

Specific scapular retraining exercises:

- Upward rotation – upper trapezius and serratus anterior
- Protraction / retraction – serratus anterior / rhomboids

Combined motor retraining exercises:

- Rotation
- Elevation (see Fig 3.31)
- Extension

Rhythmic stabilization:

- "Mirroring" – joint position sense (see Fig 3.8a-b)
- Weight bearing exercises against the wall plus medicine ball

Ongoing running programme

Maintenance of speed and power:

- drop jumps (see Fig 4.5)
- split squats

Cable exercises for trunk rotation

Technique review

Phase 4: tournament 2 – Week 4–5

The player's symptoms had settled considerably since commencing treatment and she elected to play in the second tournament. During this time, she continued to receive regular soft tissue work and practised the motor retraining exercises on a daily basis.

When she returned for further rehabilitation, she reported that her shoulder symptoms had worsened slightly with increased levels of overhead activity, but had subsided over the weekend, back to pre-tournament levels.

Phase 5: Weeks 5–8

Criteria for progression of rehabilitation: the player demonstrated good motor control of the scapulo-thoracic

and glenohumeral joints with little provocation of symptoms.

Rehabilitation goals

1. Strengthen the rotator cuff and shoulder region – commence power work
2. Improve endurance of the rotator cuff and scapular muscles
3. Maintain soft tissue extensibility and joint mobility
4. Maintain CV fitness

Rehabilitation programme

External rotation with weight / theraband (see Fig 3.34)
Compound movements for upper body strength:

- shoulder press / snatch (Fig 3.41a,b)
- cable work – overhead
- lateral flys (Fig 3.42)
- push ups with wobble board / BOSU ball (Fig 3.43a,b)

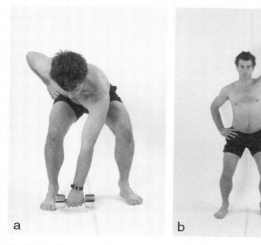

a   b

Fig 3.41 Overhead snatch with free weight showing (a) starting position and (b) finishing position.

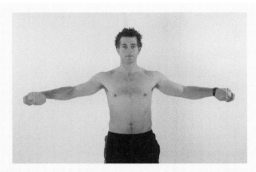

Fig 3.42 Compound movements for upper body strength.

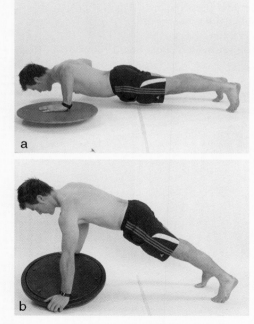

Fig 3.43 Compound movements for upper body strength – push ups using the (a) wobble board and (b) BOSU ball.

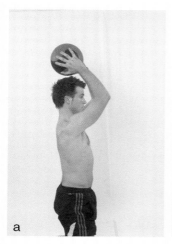 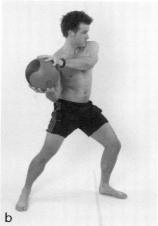

Fig 3.44 Compound movements for upper body strength: (a) overhead slams and (b) horizontal throws.

Medicine ball:

- overhead slams (Fig 3.44a)
- horizontal throws (Fig 3.44b)

Clinical commentary

This study shows that it is possible to keep an athlete competing while undergoing rehabilitation. The goals of each stage need to be very clear to everyone involved and need to be altered depending on the competition schedule.

When a player presents with an overuse problem, the clinician should use this as an opportunity to educate the player and coach about the nature of these injuries and the importance of a preventative / prehab programme.

3

Treatment and Rehabilitation

Case study – pars stress fracture

A 15-year-old schoolboy cricketer was referred by a sports physician to the physiotherapy department of a multi-disciplinary sports medicine clinic. He had presented to the physician with a 2-month history of low back pain that had gradually limited his level of sporting activity as both a fast bowler and a batsman. An MRI scan showed a right L5 pars fracture extending into the pedicle. In addition to competitive cricket, he was a keen member of his school's rugby team. His goals were to return to both cricket and rugby as quickly as possible.

Presenting problems

Symptoms and signs

- Positive extension quadrant
- Stiff thoracic and thoracolumbar spine
- Positive left straight leg raise
- Poor activation pattern of segmental multifidus
- Overactive erector spinae
- Weak / underactive gluteals
- Tight hamstrings bilaterally
- Poor deep abdominal contraction pattern
- Weak abdominals
- Tight latissimus dorsi
- Tight ITB/ vastus lateralis / hip flexors
- Tight right hip joint capsule

Problems known to be associated with the pathology

- Loss of CV fitness

Phase 1: 0–2 weeks

Rehabilitation goals

1. Protect from further injury
2. Reduce pain
3. Facilitate tissue healing
4. Maintain CV fitness

5. Improve thoracic and thoracolumbar spine mobility
6. Restore straight leg raise to normal range
7. Reduce overactivity of the erector spinae, hamstrings, latissimus dorsi, vastus lateralis and hip flexors
8. Mobilize right hip joint capsule
9. Facilitate correct deep abdominal muscle activation pattern
10. Facilitate correct activation pattern of segmental lumbar multifidus

Rehabilitation programme

Limit sporting activity – no running / rugby / cricket.

Medication for pain relief as prescribed by physician

CV fitness – cycling. Combination of steady state and interval work to stress both the aerobic and anaerobic systems.

Specific mobilization / manipulation of thoracic and thoraco-lumbar spine (Fig 3.45 and 3.46)

Mobility exercises to maintain spinal mobility

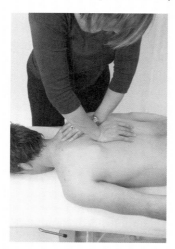

Fig 3.45 PAIVM technique to increase mobility of the thoracic spine.

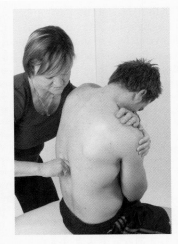

Fig 3.46 SNAG technique to increase mobility of the thoracic spine.

Specific mobilization to hip joint – extension and internal rotation

Soft tissue work – erector spinae / hamstrings / vastus lateralis and ITB / hip flexors / latissimus dorsi

Use of dry needling / IMS (www.istop.org) to reduce muscular overactivity

Neural mobilization techniques – pain free

Stretching programme for these muscles

Self massage using foam roller / spiky balls for overactive muscle groups

Phase 2: 2–6 weeks

Rehabilitation goals

Criteria for progression – correct pattern of deep abdominal and multifidus activation:

1. Maintain CV fitness
2. Maintain / improve the mobility of the thoracic spine and hip joint as required

3. Maintain SLR
4. Continue to reduce muscle overactivity / tightness as required. The need for this will be dependent upon the athlete's habitual movement patterns
5. Strengthen the abdominal muscles in an isolated fashion
6. Strengthen the gluteal muscles in an isolated fashion
7. Improve thoracic extension control

Rehabilitation programme

Continue cycling and add stair master for CV work

Mobilization / manipulation techniques with associated self mobilizing exercises for the spine and hip regions

Abdominal strengthening

Exercises to prevent excessive anterior pelvic tilt on a neutral spinal position (Fig 3.47a–c)

Exercises to improve posterior tilt and lumbar flexion (Fig 3.48)

Gluteal strengthening

Exercises to facilitate gluteal activation in the absence of lumbar spine extension (Fig 3.49a,b, see Figs 3.26 and Fig 3.28)

Home exercise programme:

- spinal mobilizing techniques
- hip joint mobilizing techniques
- neural mobilizing techniques
- self release techniques for overactive muscles
- self stretches for tight muscle regions (see Fig 3.27)
- specific stabilizing work and strength exercises

Phase 3: 6–12 weeks

Rehabilitation goals

Criteria for progression – good isolated gluteal and abdominal strength

1. Maintain CV fitness
2. Full spinal and hip ROM
3. Full flexibility of overactive / tight muscle groups

3

Treatment and Rehabilitation

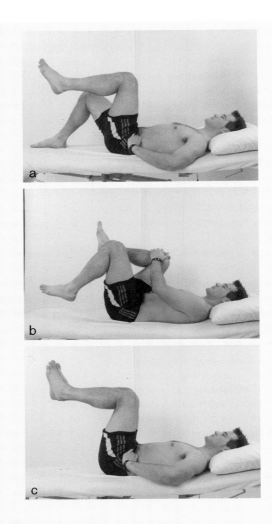

Fig 3.47 Abdominal control exercises – Sahrmann exercises level 1-3 (a–c).

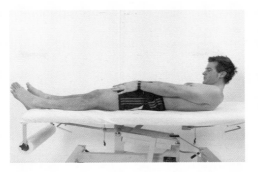

Fig 3.48 Spinal curl to increase abdominal strength.

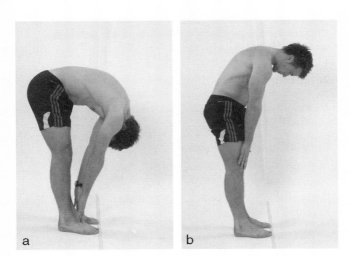

a   b

Fig 3.49 Spinal curl / uncurl showing (a) start position in hip and spinal flexion and (b) inner range position working towards hip extension with neutral spine.

4. Full neural mobility
5. Commence integrated strength activities – increase load
6. Dynamic proprioceptive training
7. Return to light jogging and restricted sport specific drills

Rehabilitation programme

Single knee bends

Squats

Bridging – single leg $\pm$ swiss ball (see Fig 3.10)

Jogging – see section "Return to running"

Progression to plyometric work – mini tramp / box jumps (see Fig 3.17)

Change of direction training – shuttle runs

Review of bowling and running technique

Phase 4: 12+ weeks

Rehabilitation goals

Criteria for progression – able to perform previous activities pain free

1. Full ROM
2. Full strength
3. Power development
4. Return to sport specific drills and restricted training and match play

Rehabilitation programme

Step ups – forward / sideways

Sprinter squats

Plyometric work for power development – bounding, hopping, hurdles (see Fig 4.9)

Jogging – to increase CV fitness

Fartlek training

Sports specific training:

- running between wickets
- bending and catching / fielding practice

Clinical commentary

The majority of bone stress injuries become asymptomatic if offloaded. The key to a comprehensive rehabilitation programme is examination of the athlete's biomechanics to determine why excessive stress is being placed on the affected region. It is essential in all cases to examine both the upper and lower kinetic chains as it may be that the biomechanical problem is located at a distance away from the injury site.

3

Treatment and Rehabilitation

Returning to play

SECTION

4

Introduction

"When can I play again?" is the million dollar question that all athletes want answered if they have been injured. The pressure on clinicians to get players back to competition as quickly as possible can be intense especially in professional sport. This pressure can come not only from the players themselves, but also from the coaching and management team and parents (in the case of young athletes). Effective goal setting that includes clinical, functional performance and sport-specific testing should be done routinely. These should be agreed from the outset and this can help to avoid any mismatch of expectation by the clinician, the athlete and members of the coaching staff and family.

There are many factors that can affect the return to training and competition, and these are not just based on the physiological aspects of healing. Psychologically, players are often not ready to return to the field even after biological healing has taken place. Most athletes will undergo a so-called 'fitness test' to see if they are fit to play. However, it is not just about the fitness test; the player should have successfully completed all the rehabilitation milestones and undertaken full participation in team practice and possibly some reserve / warm up games where practical. There may be numerous personnel involved in the rehabilitation of an injured player and each club has a different set up and processes. What is important is that in each club there is a defined protocol for return to play and it is well understood which personnel, usually the team doctor and / or physiotherapist, are responsible for the final decision that a player is fit to play. Adoption of a clear policy can help avoid any conflict during this process and help protect the player concerned. Coaching staff have been known to put pressure on a player to return to play before they are ready.

Return to play criteria should include each of the following components:

- Pathology specific
- Sport specific
- Position specific for the given sport

The late stage of rehabilitation assumes that the athlete has satisfactorily progressed through the early and middle stages of rehabilitation (see Section 3) and has no residual pain or swelling, 90% ROM and strength and good proprioception. These are the building blocks required in order to progress safely to higher demand functional performance tests, sports specific agility tests, power work and plyometric training. It is worth mentioning here that whilst athletes are continually re-assessed throughout the rehabilitation programme, in the late stage any swelling or pain induced by these activities will have an adverse effect on function and needs to be closely monitored (Fig 4.1). You don't want an athlete to get into a cycle of pain and swelling with activity. Athletes

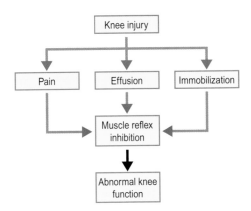

4

Returning to play

Fig 4.1 Factors contributing to muscle inhibition following joint injury.

particularly prone to this are those who have sustained articular damage following a knee or ankle injury, e.g. ACL or talar dome injury.

Finally, it is worth remembering that certain injuries, e.g. hamstring injuries, and certain sports, such as rugby, have high recurrence rates of injury. Putting a player back too soon must increase their chances of re-injury. Well defined return to play criteria that are appropriate for the player's injury, sport and position provide them and the clinician with the confidence that the player is ready to go back to full competition.

Functional performance tests

Generally, most sporting activity involves movement that requires a combination of both horizontal and vertical force production. Functional performance tests aim to simulate the forces encountered under sporting activity in a controlled environment. These tests have evolved because traditional outcome measures such as strength testing (this includes isokinetics) have only a weak to moderate relationship with functional tasks, i.e. performance. Also, strength and power has many manifestations and these can be quite specific and therefore should be tested within a functional context. Functional performance tests are highly suited for this purpose and should be incorporated into rehabilitation programmes as soon as it is safe to do so. They can be used as an objective outcome measure of progress from the middle stage right through to the end stage of the rehabilitation programme. In an ideal world athletes will have been screened for the tests that are relevant to their sport and therefore have baseline data for comparison following any injury. Functional performance tests are an indirect measure of all the following parameters:

They can be especially useful at that difficult time when the athlete has been symptom-free for a while, has full ROM, is back to running and wants to short cut the last stage of the rehabilitation phase and go straight back to playing. These tests, alongside sprint and agility drills, will often highlight the lack of full functional capacity and demonstrate to the athlete that, whilst they may feel good to go, there is still some work to do before they are ready.

A battery of functional performance tests exist (Box 4.1), from a simple single leg-hop test to the more complex and demanding cross-over hop (Fig 4.2). These may be measured for height or distance or timed, depending on the test.

Hops for distance

These are very easy to perform. Place some tape on the floor. The athlete starts with their toes just behind the tape. The distance is measured from the front of the take-off toe to the front of the landing toe. For the cross-over hop two lines of tape are placed 15 cm apart (Fig 4.3).

Timed tests

Timing systems with light sensitive gates are the best way to evaluate these. Alternatively, a stopwatch could be used. During the linear sprint test the athlete has an acceleration and deceleration box of 5 m and the sprint time is measured over 20 m (or whatever distance is most relevant) (Fig 4.4).

4

Returning to play

Box 4.1 Examples of functional performance tests

Single-leg hop   Vertical jump
Triple hop   Side jump
Stair / slope running   Shuttle runs
Figure of 8 drills   6 m timed hop
Cross-over hop   Stair hop
Vertical-squat jump   Drop jump
Linear sprint

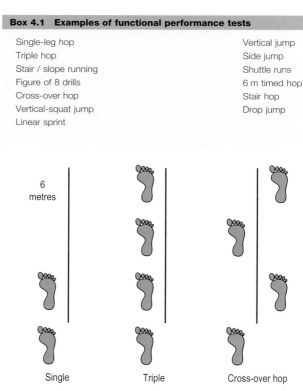

Single   Triple   Cross-over hop

Fig 4.2 Single, triple and cross-over hop for distance.

Vertical jumps

There are a variety of different vertical jump tests that can be performed and these can be evaluated using contact mat systems or force plates or the good old chalk on the finger tips and a mounted chalk board. For the vertical countermovement jump, the athlete starts on the leg to be tested with their hands on their hips. On the word "go" they quickly sink as far as necessary (around 120° knee flexion), then jump as high as possible. During the vertical squat

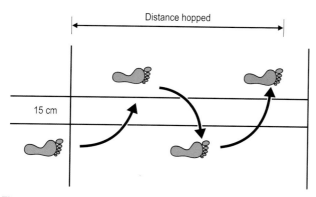

Fig 4.3 The cross-over hop for distance test.

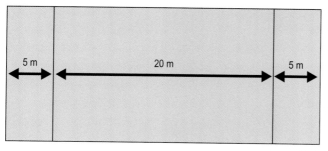

Fig 4.4 Gym or pitch layout for linear sprint test.

jump, the jump starts from a static position of 120 degrees flexion, i.e. there is no countermovement involved in this jump. Another alternative is a cyclical vertical jump. Here the athlete starts as for the countermovement jump, sinking quickly to 120 degrees flexion and then jumps as high as possible for three consecutive jumps. A drop jump where the athlete jumps off a box of predetermined height and jumps as high as possible utilizes the fast stretch–shorten cycle (SSC) typical in many sports which require rebounding phases of activity such as basketball (Fig 4.5a–c).

4

Returning to play

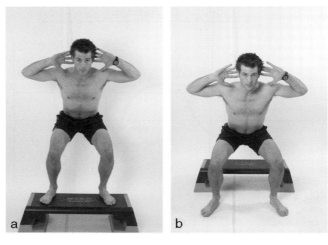

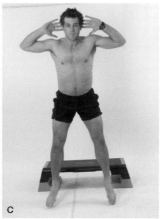

Fig 4.5 Drop jump showing (a) start, (b) mid and (c) finish positions.

The tests chosen should reflect the demands of the sport. For example, triple hops for distance and vertical jump for height would be appropriate for a basketballer where vertical and horizontal force production are equally important. A sprinter on the other hand is more interested in linear, horizontal force production.

Performing the tests

Some functional performance tests may be undertaken single or double-legged. A single-leg jump has the advantage that the limb symmetry can be calculated and used as a clinical goal if no pre-injury screening data exists for the athlete. Prior to undertaking any functional performance testing the athlete should be warmed up: a minimum warm-up routine may include 5 minutes on a stationary bike at a self-selected speed followed by dynamic stretching of the major muscle groups: Quadriceps, hamstrings and calf (gastrocnemius and soleus separately) PLUS any additional injury specific stretches 3 × 10 seconds each.

There is much debate as to how many practice and test trials should be used, and whether the mean or maximum data should be used. There is a learning and confidence effect as with any new task. I use the following protocol:

1. One or two practice trials depending on how much correction was required after the first practice.
2. Three test trials.
3. The maximum distance or height rather than the average of the three trials is used. These are performance tests, and therefore require determination of the maximum the athlete can manage.

Trials are discarded and repeated if the athlete doesn't execute the landing cleanly, without shuffling the foot, or in the case of single leg jumps, without putting the other foot down. It's not just a case of "how high" or "how far", the quality of the movement is also a key element during the execution of these tests. This is obviously a more subjective element.

4

Returning to play

For single leg tests, the limb symmetry index (LSI) can be calculated as follows:

$$\text{HOP INDEX (LSI)} = \frac{\text{INVOLVED LEG (DISTANCE or HEIGHT)}}{\text{UNINVOLVED LEG}} \times 100\%$$

A normal LSI should be greater than 85% regardless of leg dominance or sporting levels.

Functional performance tests can be used:

- As baseline tests – pre-season
- As part of a training programme
- As part of rehabilitation programme
- To monitor progress
- To identify targets for return to sport

Functional performance tests have an extensive and important role to play in both training and rehabilitation. By definition, if functional performance tests aim to truly test the functional capacity of the athlete, then there can be no such thing as a "safe" test and they can potentially exacerbate any injury. This is an important concept that both the athlete and clinician should understand, but this also comes down to the clinicians' skill of administering the right tests at the appropriate time. This paradox of using return to play evaluations may tempt the clinician into making the decision to throw the athlete back into training, because if they break down in training it is potentially perceived as unlucky, while breaking down under a test administered as part of their rehabilitation may be perceived as negligence on the part of the therapist. I suggest clinicians are not tempted to go down this route.

Sport-specific agility drills

Agility drills are used as part of training and rehabilitation and should aim to incorporate all the skills required for that specific sport. Most sports can be broken down into simple component parts. These, in turn, can be broken down into simple key elements such as linear and non-linear motion, direction of motion, speed and distance and sports-specific

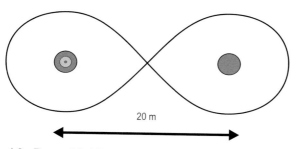

Fig 4.6 Figure of 8 drill.

skills, e.g. kicking a ball, shooting a basket, etc. These elements can initially be practised as discrete drills and then they can be combined into more complex drills that mimic manoeuvres necessary for that particular sport. Return to non-linear activities such as turning, twisting and pivoting can provide a particular challenge after ACL injury. Two useful drills here include the Figure of 8 and 45 cut or zig-zag. The Figure of 8 involves placing two cones 20 m apart and the athlete should start to run at a self-selected comfortable pace (Fig 4.6). The speed can be increased gradually. This drill aims to have the athlete turning comfortably to the right or the left. Sometimes after injury the athlete may exhibit avoidance behaviour of the activity that has previously been problematic and this may include a preference in turning. As the athlete builds up speed and confidence, the distance between the cones can be reduced by 5 m intervals until they are only 5 m apart. This graduated programme moves the athlete from making slow gentle wide turns to quick short turns in either direction.

A 45 cut or zig-zag drill is useful to see if the athlete is happy changing direction and pushing equally off both feet. The cones are set out in the gym or on the pitch as shown in Fig 4.7. The athlete has to run down the centre touching the ground on the inside of each cone with the respective foot. The foot placement should be equally firm and committed with symmetrical push-off.

4
Returning to play

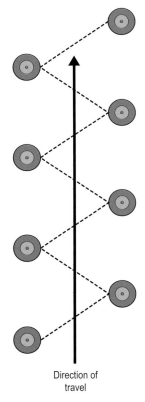

Direction of
travel

Fig 4.7 A 45 cut or zig-zag drill.

Once these drills have been completed successfully,
they can be combined into gradually more complex
combinations that replicate the sport. An example of a more
complex agility drill for a football forward is shown in
Figure 4.8.

Example progression for an agility drill:

1. Drills completed on even surface to begin with
2. Start slowly with the aim of executing the task correctly

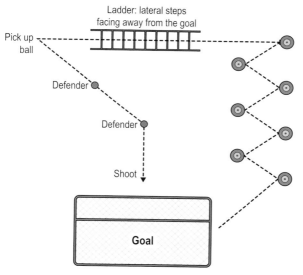

Fig 4.8 Agility drill for a central attacking forward.

3. Increase speed
4. Introduce equipment, e.g. ball
5. Move to playing surface (repeat steps 2–4)
6. Include defenders
7. Include contact

Useful web references

www.eliteathletetraining.com/Tips/Agility.aspx
www.sport-fitness-advisor.com/agilitydrills.html
www.saqinternational.com/

Plyometric training

These are covered to some extent under functional
performance tests as these two entities are not mutually

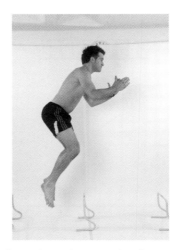

Fig 4.9 Bounding or bunny-hops over hurdles.

exclusive. However, plyometric training is specifically used to develop explosive power and should only be introduced in the late stage of the rehabilitation programme as they require a very good strength and conditioning base. Plyometric exercises apply a stretch to the muscle before the muscle contracts, and the subsequent contraction generates a greater force than if the stretch had not been applied. (This is called the stretch reflex or stretch shortening cycle (SSC).) Commonly used exercises include hopping, drop jumps (see Fig 4.5a–c) jumping and bounding (Fig 4.9).

Plyometric exercises have received considerable attention and are controversial as they have been associated with actually causing injury. They do require good conditioning of the athlete and good technique if they are to be used safely. They should only be integrated into a training / rehabilitation programme under guidance from a qualified practitioner such as the coach, strength and conditioning trainer or physiotherapist.

Top tips for plyometric exercises

1. The athlete should be well conditioned. A general yardstick seems to be at least 90% strength compared to the uninjured side.
2. An adequate warm-up should be undertaken by the athlete before starting exercise. This should include a minimum 20 minute warm-up of aerobic activity and dynamic stretching of all the relevant muscle groups.
3. Good landing technique must be emphasised – "soft knee", to absorb the high forces with good dynamic valgus alignment, i.e. the knee should drive over the 2nd toe.
4. Pick the right type of exercise for the sport.
5. Start with smaller jumps before progressing to higher ones.
6. Adequate rest times should occur between reps and sessions.
7. Avoid using uneven and hard training surfaces.
8. STOP the athlete exercising on the slightest hint of any niggle, pull or pain.

Useful web references

www.sport-fitness-advisor.com/plyometricexercises.html

www.sportsmedicine.about.com/od/sampleworkouts/a/Plyometrics.htm

www.myfit.ca/exercisedatabase/plyometrics.asp?type=Sport%20Specific%20Exercises

4

Returning to play

Additional power training

Overload principles apply to power training and there are many ways athletes can develop power using a variety of different methods of resistance including Olympic lifts such as power cleans (Fig 4.10a–c). Sand / uphill / parachutes or

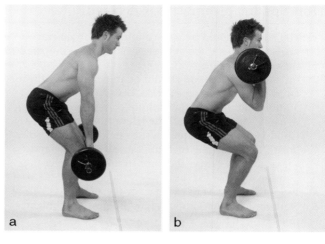

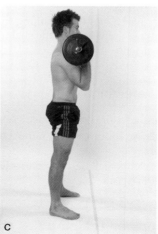

Fig 4.10 Power cleans (a) start, (b) mid and (c) finish position.

bungee resistance, can be used to develop explosive running, bungee cords for explosive jumping.

The "fitness test"

Everyone is familiar with the so-called "fitness test" which is often advocated in the media as being the test a player has to pass before they are able to play again following an injury. This "test" has less to do with physiological status and more with satisfying a number of criteria, many of which will have been achieved during the progress of the rehabilitation. These criteria may vary depending on the sport, the position played and the injury. Little has been written on what are the best / most appropriate criteria when considering return to play practices. Table 4.1 shows examples of fitness test elements used in a survey of return to play practices in elite and club level rugby union in New Zealand. The list represents the rank order of importance considered by the personnel responsible for return to play decisions.

4

Returning to play

Table 4.1 Fitness test elements used for return to play assessment in rugby union

1. Ability to complete position-specific drills
2. Injury-specific tests
3. Sprint tests (acceleration / deceleration)
4. Walk / jog / run patterns
5. Tackling drills
6. Scrummaging activities
7. Agility speed tests
8. Jumping / hopping tests
9. Lifting drills
10. Down and up drill
11. Push-up variations
12. Bleep test or 3 km run

I think it is fair to say that the end stage phase has traditionally been the least well understood and practised phase of rehabilitation. With the increase in numbers of strength and conditioning trainers now employed in professional sport the responsibility for this phase has gradually been taken over by these professionals and the therapist will hand over the care of the athlete once they have reached this phase. However, in clubs and sport settings where this back-up is not available, the therapist will need either to take the player through this phase or, at the very least, be able to advise what the player needs to do before returning to full competition. The latter is particularly important for clinic-based therapists. This section has highlighted those key elements that need to be considered in order to return the player to the competitive arena without fear of re-injury.

Comprehensive player management

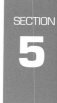

SECTION

5

Travelling with a team

International events and major games can be the pinnacle of a physiotherapist's career with a team and can be a very rewarding experience. They can also provide nightmares that can easily be avoided by following some simple do's and don'ts. This list is by no means exhaustive but will give you some ideas of what to look for if you are facing your first big trip. Of course it depends on what other personnel you have around you; you might be travelling as part of a large squad with a big medical team, in which case you will have plenty of support. More often than not you will be the only "medical" person with little to call on in the event of an emergency.

Preparation

The basic premise when travelling with a team is to be completely self-sufficient. You then won't fall short unless there is an emergency and you should plan contingency for these. **Preparation is the key to success.**

Find out as much as you can well before you are due to set off. If you are not involved in a recce prior to the event, give a list questions about the facilities and equipment available at the hotel, training and competition venues to someone who is.

Basic checklist

- Transport available
- Food: sample menus/portions/timing
- Hydration: water/isotonic drinks
- Ice
- Treatment plinths (adjustable or fixed)
- Dedicated space to set up own medical/treatment area
- Emergency back-up
- Specialist referral ± diagnostics, e.g. blood tests and imaging

(See also Section 1: Know your location.)

What to take with you?

Take everything you anticipate needing. Even if you are visiting a country with access to good medical supplies, you will not have time to go out sourcing and shopping for these. Competition is an intense time and your focus should be on the athletes. Make sure any electrical equipment has had the appropriate checks, that you have extension leads and the right adaptors for the country in which you are competing.

Check whether any vaccinations or anti-malarial medications are required, together with any certification necessary.

 Make sure you have a current passport with at least 6 months until its expiry date and check whether a visa is required – there is nothing more embarrassing than arriving at the airport to find it has expired. The Foreign and Commonwealth Office web site is a useful source of information for health and travel regulations worldwide when travelling from the UK (www.fco.gov.uk/en).

You will possibly be travelling with athletes you are familiar with and whose medical and musculoskeletal history is known to you. But you could also be covering a team you don't know or are relatively unfamiliar with. In the latter scenario it is very useful to try and gain as much knowledge about the athletes beforehand and for them to meet you as well. Get in touch with their regular clinician (if they have one) to find more information. Try and attend some training sessions prior to departing and / or shadow the regular clinician. I have never travelled with a squad of athletes that have been completely injury-free; it is therefore useful to know the problems you are going to have to deal with.

If possible, get to meet the rest of the team beforehand as well; this includes the team manager, coaching and any other medical and support staff. It is important that you and everyone else are clear as to exactly what your role is during your time with the squad. Likewise it is essential that you understand the role of all other members of the team. Don't forget, you may be asked to help with any

5

Comprehensive player management

injuries of the non-athletes in your team – be prepared for this. See also Section 1: Know your team.

Travelling

Dealing with jet lag and time zones

It is recommended that the athletes start to prepare roughly a week beforehand (for large time differences) and gradually changes their sleep patterns to adjust to the country where they are going. Melatonin and sleeping tablets go in and out of fashion but are best avoided unless an athlete is used to taking them. On arrival, try and get everyone into the local time as soon as possible. Remember that the effects of jet lag are worse travelling east compared to west. After a long haul flight, do not allow the athletes to train too hard for the first few days. A general rule of thumb is to allow one day's recovery for each time zone change.

   Be prepared for travel delays with food and medication. Ensure athletes have a warm jumper / fleece in their hand luggage. Planes can often be quite cold.

Tips for flying

- Reset your watch to local time
- Make sure you take any special foods / medicines in the cabin with you
- Drink plenty of fluids (no alcohol)
- Get up and move regularly – do heel raises

During the event

See Section 1 for details to check at local venues. It is worth investigating referrals to local specialists if required. There is normally a medical contact or liaison officer for the local organizing committee who can answer any queries.

Clinic set-up

Ideally, there should be a dedicated room in the accommodation to set up a clinic. However, many times when space is at a premium or it is too costly to do this, your bedroom doubles as a clinic space – this is not ideal, but it does happen and you have to be flexible in these situations and provide a professional service regardless of the scenarios you may be faced with. Do you take your own treatment tables? Yes, if you can. I have been to tournaments where provision of a treatment table was promised, only to find there were not enough for the number of clinicians and athletes. I would recommend a minimum of one portable plinth per clinician. There is a wide variety available on the market and my personal preference is a light plinth, with a lifting end (so the player can sit up) and adjustable height.

Hours of work and access

Be clear about your hours of work and where and how the athletes can access you. A timetable outside the treatment room of available appointment slots that the athletes can sign up for normally works well. A mobile contact number should also be on the door so the players can contact you when you are not there. If you are working with a team, access to you is straightforward – you follow the team. If it is an individual sport, e.g. swimming or athletics, depending on how many clinicians there are you will allocate your time accordingly between the hotel and competition venue to suit the warm-up and race times of the athletes. Arrange your schedule so you can accommodate all the athletes as necessary but also give yourself some downtime as well. You don't want to burn out halfway through a competition because you have been doing 16 hour days. How late is it reasonable to work? This will vary depending on the competition schedule and you have to be flexible to accommodate this. Don't forget to allocate time to non-treatment activities such as paperwork, liaising with other medical staff, attending meetings, etc.

Illness

Athletes are in continual close proximity, often sharing accommodation, and any cold can quickly travel round an entire squad. Additionally, travel in certain countries carries

5

Comprehensive player management

a higher risk of gastrointestinal problems and travellers' diarrhoea.

Any of these illnesses can have a devastating effect on a squad. The key here is prevention.

Tips for staying healthy in "at risk" countries

- Wash your hands regularly with alcohol gel especially before eating
- Only drink bottled water
- Never add ice to any drinks
- Drink from straws that are wrapped rather than directly from a bottle or can.
- Avoid salads, raw fruit and vegetables

It is essential to discuss these tips with the athletes, especially the importance of hand washing. I always travel with a packet of "wet wipes" as well as the hand gel, as in some places access to good hand washing facilities may be difficult.

Immediate isolation and management of any affected team or team member is essential to avoid cross infection.

Communication

You need to establish an effective communication system, especially if you are working at an event where there are multiple sites. This may be by walkie-talkie or mobile, but make sure you have the contact numbers of all the team.

Documentation

It is a real challenge working at any venue as opposed to a clinic based situation. Section 1 includes an easy form that can be used in a first aid situation; however, there should be a standard format whereby any intervention / consultation is recorded. This is a statutory requirement, for your and the athlete's protection. Continuity of care for

athletes who spend a lot of time travelling from one
training camp / competition to another, often with
different support teams, is a challenge. It is often difficult
for the medical team to monitor and assess the athlete's
progress. Paper report systems have largely been superseded
by injury databases such as Injury Zone, a web-based
database through which clinicians can access an athlete's
information anytime and anywhere.

After the event

Once you have arrived back home, your job is rarely
finished. Any follow-up needs to be managed. This might
include sourcing treatment or diagnostics local to the
athlete. You may be required to write a debrief report,
including an evaluation of the service provided and any
recommendations for future events.

Patient confidentiality

Most healthcare professionals involved in the care of
athletes are bound by a code of professional conduct and,
as such, have a duty of confidentiality to the athlete in
their care. The duty of confidentiality means that no
personal information obtained in a consultation between
the athlete and a healthcare professional can be passed on
to any third party without the athlete's consent.

Physiotherapists in particular spend a lot of time with
players and may become party to a lot of personal
information from players in the course of consultations and
treatment. They quickly get a reputation within a club as
someone the players can trust or as someone who they know
will relay any information directly back to the coaches. In
the latter scenario, players may choose to limit the
information supplied during the course of the consultation,
which may result in less than optimal management. It could
potentially put the athlete at risk, if the athlete is trying to

"play injured" and is being untruthful about the problem. Additionally, if there is a lack of trust between the healthcare professional within a squad or club, the athlete may seek treatment outside the club. Neither of these scenarios is good for the athlete or the team.

Ideally, and this is where continuity in any club is important, there is an understanding of these issues and what the code of conduct is between the management and coaches, the medical support staff and the athletes. Be aware that it takes time and effort to develop a trusting relationship between all parties.

This might all seem very straightforward; however, conflicts can and do arise. Personal information gleaned in a consultation may not relate just to an injury or illness; it could be other information that could affect the player's performance, for example, taking banned substances, excessive drinking, etc. How would you deal with a scenario like this? What would you do if a player comes to see you with an injury and tells you not to let the management know as he wants to play this coming weekend? It will probably be in the player's best interests that the management are aware of the problem for various reasons: you might want to take the player out of training to do some specific testing, you might want to agree a strategy to manage this injury which may include modification to the normal training (which is not easy to do without the management's knowledge), or there may be some reorganization with the starting line up or substitutes named if it is known a player is not 100% fit. You also want to protect the player from any further damage which could have more serious ramifications. If the management are aware then they can also be on the lookout for any signs the player might be struggling. There are normally many reasons that can be used to persuade a player that it makes sense for the management to be aware of any problems, primarily for the protection of the players themselves.

A physiotherapist employed by a club may feel their loyalty is to the club and may feel duty-bound to report these issues to their employer. Additionally, some managers or coaches have an expectation that they should know everything about their players. It is important that the management are aware of the clinician's responsibilities regarding confidentiality. Ideally this should all be achieved in a non-confrontational manner and established **before** a crisis arises, as this will always complicate matters. Players are always suspicious if there is a change of management in a club and they arrive with their own "back room" team. Healthcare professionals who follow the management team may feel indebted to them for their jobs and see their duty as being to the management team rather than the athlete. Commercial and media pressures are also a consideration in professional sport and the importance of an impending game may bring additional pressures on the medical team to get an athlete back playing.

Good and effective working dynamics between the management team, medical team and athletes are imperative for the optimal management and protection of the athlete. There are many good clinicians who can treat athletes perfectly well but struggle to manage the dynamics of their working environment. A thorough understanding of issues surrounding patient confidentiality will help the clinician avoid any potential conflicts within their practice. As always, this should be combined with a dose of discretion and diplomacy on behalf of the clinician.

There are many consensus and position statements written on this subject and I include one from the British Olympic Association as an example for further reading. This position statement also contains an example of an athlete consent form (Fig 5.1)

British Olympic Association (2000). The British Olympic Association's position statement on athlete confidentiality. British Journal of Sports Medicine 34:71-72.

5

Comprehensive player management

ATHLETE CONSENT FORM

I agree/do not agree to relevant details from consultations, tests or treatment undertaken by

.... in ....
(year/season)

being released to...*(e.g. coach/performance director/member of support staff)*

I realise that refusal to give consent for the release of the details will not affect my access to medical care, treatment or testing. It cannot be guaranteed that others will not use this refusal of consent in relation to selection.

Consent can be withdrawn at any time, and only notice of its withdrawal will be released to those specified above.

I have read the above notes on informed consent and fully understand them.

Signed... Date..
(to be signed also by parent or guardian for those under 18)

Fig 5.1 BOA Athlete consent form.

Drugs in sport

Cheating in sport is attractive to those athletes who want to win at any cost. Equally, an athlete struggling to overcome an injury may be tempted to use illegal means to enhance their recovery. Unfortunately, there have been too many episodes in recent times of high profile athletes abusing the system and their bodies. The World Anti-Doping Agency (WADA) is recognized by the International Olympic

Committee (IOC) and many other International Federations as the organization responsible for promoting, co-ordinating and monitoring the fight against doping in sport in all its forms. WADA produce a list of prohibited and restricted drugs in sport, which is revised on an annual basis (www. wada-ama.org).

Ignorance is no longer a defence for testing positive and athletes should be taught that they are responsible for any substance ingested. The athlete should be aware of the list and should have access to an appropriately qualified doctor or pharmacist to ask advice regarding any prescribed or non-prescribed medicine. This also applies to all off the shelf supplements as some of these have shown to contain substances that could lead to a positive test. Athletes cannot be certain of the quality or contamination of such products. Each batch would have to be tested to make sure it was clean. The 2010 Prohibited List (International Standard) came into effect on the 1 January 2010 and can be found on the WADA website.

The list is compiled under four different sections:

- Prohibited substances
- Prohibited methods
- Substances and methods prohibited in competition
- Substances prohibited in particular sports

Prohibited substances

- S1 Anabolic agents
- S2 Peptide hormones, growth factors and related substances
- S3 Beta-2 agonists
- S4 Hormone antagonists and modulators
- S5 Diuretics and other masking agents

Prohibited methods

- M1 Enhancement of oxygen transfer (blood doping)
- M2 Chemical and physical manipulation (tampering with the sample)
- M3 Gene doping

Blood doping involves the removal and storage of the athlete's whole blood or blood products. This is then reintroduced into the athlete's system at a later date when the circulating volume has naturally recovered, thereby boosting the red cell count in order to improve performance. This practice has largely been superseded by the use of erythropoietin (EPO) in endurance sports such as cycling and cross-country skiing.

Tampering with the sample can fall into one of three categories:

1. *In vivo*: imbibing a substance prior to micturition that will mask a positive test, e.g. diuretics
2. *In vitro*: adding substances to the sample after micturition to prevent detection
3. Sample substitution, whereby a clean substitute sample (from the athlete or donor) is provided via a concealed source

Substances prohibited in competition

Stimulants
Narcotics
Cannabinoids
Gluticosteroids

Alcohol is banned in competition in certain sports such as archery and modern pentathlon. Beta-blockers are banned during competition in sports that require a steady hand as they slow the heart rate and reduce tremor. They are banned in sports such as archery, snooker and shooting events.

In- and out-of-competition drug testing is now well established and high performance athletes can be expected to be tested many times during their career. Out-of-competition testing has been particularly controversial and athletes have fallen foul of the "missed 3 tests and you are out" rule. Recent changes to the "whereabouts rule" should make the out-of-competition testing easier for the athletes, trainers and testers.

Athletes, like all of us, may suffer an illness or condition that requires them to take particular medication. If the medication is on the Prohibited List, a Therapeutic Use Exemption (TUE) may give that athlete the authorization to take the needed medicine.

The criteria for granting a TUE are:

- The athlete would experience significant health problems without taking the prohibited substance or method
- The therapeutic use of the substance would not produce significant enhancement of performance
- There is no reasonable therapeutic alternative to the use of the otherwise prohibited substance or method

A TUE can be obtained from the athlete's national anti-doping organization or their international federation. WADA are not responsible for issuing TUEs but may be involved in any appeal.

Any of the medical team may be involved with the testing procedure and both the athlete and anyone accompanying them during a test should be fully aware of the correct procedure. The latest testing procedures for blood and urine testing can be found on the UK Anti-Doping Agency (UKAD) website (www.ukad.org.uk).

Global Drug Reference Online (www.globaldro.com) is a useful website athletes or the support team can search for brand name drugs to see what their status is and whether an exemption is required. The same brands can vary in their contents depending on where in the world they are sold, so do not assume that a comparable brand bought in a different country is safe. This website will also check a limited number of countries depending on where you bought the medication, including the USA. So, an inhaler used by an athlete in the UK which contains no banned substances may not be the same when bought in a different country. The website can provide this information to athletes and clinicians.

The current drives both nationally and internationally aim to educate the athletes to be clean and responsible.

Hot climates

If athletes are due to train or compete in a hot climate they will need to acclimatize to the heat to ensure their performance is not affected. Athletes are more likely to become dehydrated in this environment and this will compound the effect of the heat and reduce performance.

Advice for athletes on coping with heat

- A minimum of 7–10 days' heat acclimatization is advisable before competition
- If possible, try to get access to a heat chamber before going to a hot climate, together with good advice on its use
- During competition and training be aware of symptoms such as headache, nausea, dizziness and lack of co-ordination. These may be an indication of dehydration or heat stress
- You may need to modify your warm-up so that you do not overheat. If possible, warm-up in an air-conditioned environment
- Stay in the shade (if possible) until immediately before your event
- Reduce your body temperature after exercise by finding shade or an air-conditioned room
- Your heart rates for equivalent exercise will be increased until you acclimatize to the heat. You may need to adapt your training to account for this
- Consult a doctor if you have an illness that could be dehydrating such as a fever, upper respiratory tract infection or diarrhoea and sickness. It may be necessary to reduce or stop training
- Room temperatures should not be set too low as frequent changes from high to low temperatures may cause upper respiratory problems such as a sore throat, cough and runny nose
- Keep cool at night time so that you sleep well. Do not turn off the air-conditioning. Doing so will not help you to acclimatize
- CARRY DRINKS WITH YOU AT ALL TIMES
  You can quickly become dehydrated
  if you get stuck somewhere
  and cannot get a drink

  British Olympic Association Guidelines (1993) The Traveling Athlete. Olympic Medical Institute.

If athletes have to be out in the sun, ensure they:

- Minimize the amount of time they are under direct exposure
- Cover up (clothes) any skin that doesn't need to be exposed
- Apply waterproof sun block to any exposed areas prior to going outside. Sport blocks designed for sailors are not oily, don't weep into the eyes and don't cause them to lose their grip
- Re-apply regularly as necessary
- Wear a hat and sunglasses
- Use electrolyte drinks in addition to water

Additionally, make sure that shade is available

Thermoregulation is the ability to maintain relative thermal homeostasis between heat loss and heat gain. Thermoregulation plays an important role in cellular metabolism and failure to maintain this homeostasis can lead to cellular ion fluxes, changes in pH and denaturation of proteins.

Exertional heat illness can manifest itself as muscle cramping, heat exhaustion or, in the worst case, exertional heatstroke. Any athlete engaged in prolonged intense activity can suffer from heat illness and whilst it occurs more frequently in hot and humid climates, it can occur in cool conditions as well. A full description of exertional heat illness can be found in the ACSM position statement (www. acsm.org)

American College of Sports Medicine (ACSM) (2007) Exertional heat illness during training and competition. Medicine & Science in Sports and Exercise 556-572.

Cold climates

Cold weather *per se* does not present the same problems as exercising in the heat, and any physiological adaptations are far more subtle. Athletes involved in winter sports or subjected to exercise in a cold climate are at risk from

5

Comprehensive player management

frostbite (if the tissue temperature falls below 0°C) and hypothermia. Any exposed skin and hands and feet are more likely to get frostbite. This is associated with an initial onset of numbness and then the skin turns a waxy white colour. Removal of any wet clothing and slow re-warming is recommended. This process can be very painful. Prevention is the key here, and clothing is very important. Wear multiple layers where possible and make sure the material can wick; wet clothing will have a significant effect on body temperature. Gloves and head cover will also reduce heat loss.

Exercise induced bronchospasm (EIB) is exacerbated in cold temperatures. The prevalence of EIB in winter athletes has been shown to be much higher in sports such as figure skating (35%) and cross country skiing (28%) compared to the general population (5-10%). Symptoms can include wheezing, coughing, a feeling of tightness in the chest, difficulty in breathing and excess mucus production. Treatment for EIB is an inhaled beta-2 agonist such as Ventolin or a corticosteroid such as Becotide or a combination of these such as Symbicort. These drugs are on the Prohibited List (see Drugs in sport) and athletes now need to provide evidence of the need for medication to treat EIB. This can be achieved through a bronchodilator or bronchoprovocation challenge.

American College of Sports Medicine (2006) Prevention of cold injuries during exercise. Medicine & Science in Sports and Exercise 2012-2029.

Hydration

It is well established that athletes should be hydrated in order to achieve optimal performance. I am therefore constantly surprised by the number of athletes, and this includes professional rugby and football players, that routinely train and compete in a dehydrated state.

Advice to athletes – how to check if you are dehydrated

1. Check the colour of your urine against a urine colour chart
2. Weigh yourself. Check your weight before and after exercise to see how much water you have lost through sweating. Ideally this should be done naked as sweat will get trapped in clothes and this will underestimate the amount of water loss
3. Urine osmolality and specific gravity can be checked using more complex equipment. Athletes who have science support will have access to this

Advice to athletes – avoiding dehydration

Check your hydration status each morning – urine and body weight

1 kg of body mass = 1 litre of water

< 2% BW = dehydration = 10% drop in performance

Drink 1.5 litres of water for every kg of weight loss

Drink 600-1200 ml/hour during exercise

If you are thirsty, you are already dehydrated

The more humid it is, the more likely you are to get dehydrated

One word of caution: an excessive intake of water during endurance events can lead to exercise-induced hyponatraemia, which is a drop in plasma sodium. This is a rare but potentially life-threatening condition. Symptoms become progressively worse depending on the amount of sodium loss but can include headaches, vomiting, disorientation and confusion, swollen hands, wheezy breathing leading to seizure, collapse and death.
American College of Sports Medicine (2007) Exercise and fluid replacement. Medicine & Science in Sports and Exercise 377-390.

5

Comprehensive player management

Glossary

A&E	Accident and Emergency
ABC	Airway, breathing and circulation
Abd	Abduction
AC	Acromioclavicular
ACL	Anterior cruciate ligament
ACPSM	Association of Chartered Physiotherapists in Sports Medicine
ACSM	American College of Sports Medicine
AP	Anterior–posterior
ATFL	Anterior talofibular ligament
BASEM	British Association of Sports and Exercise Medicine
BOA	British Olympic Association
Ca	Cancer
CAI	Chronic ankle instability
CECS	Chronic exertional compartment syndrome
CFL	Calcaneofibular ligament
CSP	Chartered Society of Physiotherapy
CT	Computed tomography
CV	Cardiovascular
DF	Dorsiflexion
EAB	Elastic adhesive bandage
ECRB	Extensor carpi radialis brevis
EIB	Exercise-induced asthma
EPO	Erythropoietin
ER	External rotation
Exs	Exercises
Ext	External
FAI	Femoroacetabular impingement
HI	Head injury

IFSP	International Federation of Sports Physiotherapy
IMS	Intramuscular stimulation
IR	Internal rotation
ITB	Iliotibial band
IVF	Intervertebral foramen
GHJ	Glenohumeral joint
GTN	Glyceryl trinitrate
LA	Local anaesthetic
LBP	Low back pain
Lat	Latissimus
LCL	Lateral collateral ligament
LF	Lateral flexion
MCL	Medial collateral ligament
MCP	Metacarpophalangeal
MRA	Magnetic resonance arthrography
MRI	Magnetic resonance imaging
MT	Musculo-tendinous
MTP	Metatarsophalangeal
MTSS	Medial tibial stress syndrome
MWM	Mobilization with movement
NAD	No abnormality detected
NAG	Natural apophyseal glides
NOF	Neck of femur
NOI	Neuro Orthopaedic Institute
NSAID	Non-steroidal anti-inflammatory drug
NWB	Non weight-bearing
OA	Osteoarthritis
PAIVM	Passive accessory intervertebral movement
Pec	Pectoralis
PCL	Posterior cruciate ligament
P/F	Patellofemoral
PFPS	Patellofemoral pain syndrome
PKE	Passive knee extension
PPIVM	Passive physiological intervertebral movement
PWB	Partial weight-bearing
R=L	Right equals left
ROM	Range of movement
Rot	Rotation

RTP	Return to play
SNAG	Sustained natural apophyseal glides
T/F	Tibiofemoral
TFCC	Triangular fibrocartilage complex
TUE	Therapeutic Use Exemption
UKAD	UK Anti-Doping Agency
ULNPT	Upper limb neural provocation test
US	Ultrasound
VAS	Visual analogue scale
VMO	Vastus medialis obliquus
WAD	Whiplash associated disorder
WADA	World Anti-Doping Agency
WFATT	World Federation of Athletic Training and Therapy

Index

NB: Page numbers in *italics* refer to boxes, figures and tables.

A

Neurological examination, 109,
110, 117
Neurological pain, 138
Neuromuscular components,
169–170
Non steroidal anti-inflammatory
drugs (NSAIDS)
ankle sprain, 180
shoulder impingement, 223,
224
Nordic drills, 193–194, *193*

O

'OAdjuster' brace, 175
Ober's test, *85*, 86, 89
Objective examination, 40
see also specific injuries
Observation, 44, 117
Oedema, 155–156, 157, 158
'Off loading' braces, 175
One leg standing exercise, 128,
128
Open chain pattern, 172
Osteoarthritis, 175
Osteochondrosis, 140
Overhead slams, 229, *229*
Overhead snatch, *227*
Overload principles, 168,
253–255
Oxford scale of muscle strength,
168

P

Painful movement, 165
Parathyroid hormone, 92
Pars interarticularis stress
fracture, 127–129
Pars stress fracture, case study,
230–237

Passive accessory intervertebral
movements (PAIVMs),
118, 133, 141, *231*
Passive knee extension (PKE)
test, *77*
Passive physiological
intervertebral movements
(PPIVMs), 118, 141
Passive stretch, quadriceps, 75,
76, *76*
Patella tendinopathy, 87–89
Patellofemoral/anterior knee
pain, 84–87, 89, 116
Peripheral joints, 41–46
Personal histories, 259
Phagocytosis, 152
Physical examination,
117–118
Physiological processes, 149
Pivot shift test, 80, *80*
Placement tasks, 172–174
Plank holds, 220, *221*
Plantar fasciitis, 116
Plantar nerves, 116
Plyometric exercise, 210
ankle sprain, 186, *187*
drills, 169–170
training, 251–253
Posterior cruciate ligament
(PCL), 83–84
Posture, 135
Power cleans, 253–255, *254*
Power training, 253–255
Practice trials, 247
PRICE (mnemonic), 50
ankle sprain, 180
cervical zygopophyseal
(facet) joint, 133
costovertebral joint sprain,
143
hamstring injury, 78